AUTOPHAGY & INTERMITTENT FASTING

2 BOOKS IN 1

How to Detox your Body, Live Healthier and Longer trough Diet, Fasts and Excercise. A Practical Guide on How to Activate Autophagy Safely

Patricia Cook

Table of Content

Autophagy

Learn HOW TO ACTIVATE AUTOPHAGY SAFELY Through Intermittent Fasting, Exercise and DIET. A Practical GUIDE to DETOX Your Body and BOOST Your Energy

Introduction

Did you know that our forefathers did not have access to half as much food we have access to these days? Yet they were strong, healthy, agile, and lived long lives. They were not susceptible to many diseases like cancer, diabetes, and obesity, which are now the order of the day. They were able to trek long distances, fight off wild animals, and climb rocks without much adverse effect on their health.

What was the secret to their health?

They did not eat abundantly like we do today. Food was scarce then, since they had to hunt and go about picking fruits. It was easy for their bodies to get access to the important nutrients at the right quantities. This way, their body systems could easily alternate between the fed and fasted states. This resulted in tremendous health benefits, benefits that are alien to many people today.

These days, there's food around every corner. Food is so much in abundance that we do not give our body the chance to switch to a fasted state. To make matters worse, unhealthy and fast foods are lurking everywhere. This conditions our body for a variety of diseases like heart disease, cancer, and diabetes.

This is not surprising, as we do not give our body the chance to reap the tremendous health benefits that come with being in the fasted state. Constant eating disturbs the natural balance of the body, hence we rob ourselves of exploring the self healing capacity of our body. It is not surprising that we now have to deal with many adverse health conditions that were alien to our forefathers.

If you try to return the body to the natural state of equilibrium, however, where it alternates between the feasting and the fasted state, there are many health benefits you will reap. One of these processes is the phenomenon called autophagy.

Autophagy is a topic that has been subjected to countless studies and experimentations from medical experts, fitness experts, dietitians, and many other health related professionals all around the globe since the 1960s. The study of autophagy is mainly concerned with the metabolism of the different cells of the human body and how they renew their dysfunctional counterparts. Understanding of its apparent effect on human physiology has advanced rapidly since the 90s, after the study of yeast uncovered the working process of autophagy. Just a few years back, there was a breakthrough in autophagy studies which bought it to mainstream attention again. These were the results of the studies of Japanese researcher Yoshinori Ohsumi (Ohsumi, 2014).

There is a direct correlation between autophagy and fasting, as the long breaks between the fasts promote the energy levels of the cells of our body, which will be discussed in further detail later on in the book.

It is high time you quit seeing your ancestors as some superior yet unattainable beings. They were normal men and women that were disciplined enough to equip their bodies with the necessary resources to explore the benefits of autophagy.

Their major occupation was hunting and fruit gathering, hence their lifestyle made it easy for them to fast and exercise. Unlike today, where our digestive system has no chance to rest and a sedentary lifestyle is what many people are used to.

Take this book as a manual to give you a reorientation concerning your approach and relation to food. We will explore the concept of autophagy and how you can benefit from it. There is a chapter dedicated to the benefits of autophagy as well as the concepts of macro and micro autophagy. More importantly, we will explore how to activate the autophagy process in your body safely through fasting.

All in all, get ready for a unique change that will make your body resistant and immune to disease and also help you enjoy long, full, healthy years.

It is possible, with the concept of autophagy!

Chapter 1:
Autophagy: What It Is

The word autophagy takes its roots from the ancient Greek word αὐτόφαγος (autophagocytosis), which translates to self-devouring or self-cannibalism, but within the cells of a living organism. But don't start panicking; autophagy is actually a healthy process of maintaining and replenishing the important organs that we rely on to operate in our day-to-day life. Just like machinery and other objects around us, our body cells also decay and become incapable of functioning properly. When this occurs, it becomes necessary to replenish those dead or useless cells with new ones, and this is where autophagy kicks in and helps the body.

The discovery and progress of the studies on autophagy originally started way back in 1963, when a Belgian biochemist named Christian De Duve started his studies on the function of lysosomes which led to the discovery of autophagy. But it wasn't until the 90s that autophagy became more understandable once scientists managed to finally grasp the mechanism of autophagy and how it affects the human body. Even to this day, though a lot of light has been shed on the mechanisms of autophagy, how autophasogome, the organ responsible for autophagic cycle, is formed still remains a mystery.

There are 3 main types of autophagy - macroautophagy, microautophagy, and CMA (chaperone-mediated autophagy). Macroautophagy is the main autophagic pathway of the autophagic process and deals with delivering cytoplasmic components to the lysosome, while microautophagy deals with dissolving that cargo into the autophagosome formed during the autophagic process. Autophagy occurs in the body by converting the discarded and useless cell parts into amino acids. Here is a basic discussion of macroautophagy, microautophagy, and chaperone-mediated autophagy for the sake of understanding these elements. The first 2 two elements of autophagy will be discussed further in Chapter 3 of the book.

Macroautophagy

Among the three types of autophagy, macroautophagy is the main and most important process or pathway. The primary use of macroautophagy is to get rid of non-functioning cell organelles or proteins that remain unused in the body. Macroautophagy can again be divided into two types, namely bulk macroautophagy and selective macroautophagy. The difference between these two is just as their names suggest. At first, it was thought that macroautophagy did not distinguish which damaged organelles to get rid of and was a bulk process, but later studies showed that despite its bulk removal process, there is selective macroautophagy which involves the removal of certain organelles such as mitophagy, lipophagy, pexophagy, chlorophagy, etc.

The process of macroautophagy is quite simple. At first, the organelles that need to be eradicated are engulfed by the phagophore. This results in the formation of a double membrane around the organelle known as the autophagosome. Once formed, the autophagosome travels to lysosome through the cytoplasm, where it fuses with the lysosome. The lysosome then releases acidic lysosomal hydrolase which degrades the contents of the autophagosome, thus completing the process.

Microautophagy

Unlike macroautophagy, the process of microautophagy involves the lysosome directly engulfing cytoplasmic materials. This process is possible because of the inward folding of lysosomal membrane, which is called invagination. Microautophagy can also be divided into two types, which are selective and non-selective microautophagy. Selective microautophagy can be observed mostly in yeast cells. Again, there are three types of selective microautophagy, namely micropexophagy, piecemeal microautophagy, and micromitophagy. On the other hand, non-selective microautophagy can be observed in all types of eukaryotic cells.

It is important to note that although macro and microautophagy are two different processes, both of them are necessary to recycle nutrients under starvation.

Chaperone-mediated Autophagy

CMA for short is a very complex form of autophagy and is very specific in nature. This type of autophagy requires the protein that needs to be degraded to be recognized by an Hsc70 containing complex. This simply means that the protein must contain a recognition site that will allow it to be bonded to an Hsc70 complex. Once bonded, the protein and the complex will form a CMA-substrate complex which will travel to the lysosome. Once there, the CMA complex will be recognized and will be allowed to enter the cell. Upon entering, the protein will get unfolded and will be moved across the lysosome membrane, degrading it in the process. The difference between CMA and the other types of autophagy is its extremely selective nature.

History of Autophagy

The first recorded observation of autophagy was at the Rockefeller Institute by Keith R. Porter, a Canadian-American cell biologist and his student Thomas Ashford (Ashford, 1962).

In 1962 while observing rat liver cells, they reported that the number of lysosomes increased after the addition of glucagon, which is a peptide hormone produced by the cells in the pancreas. They also observed that other cell organelles such as mitochondria, which is also called the powerhouse of the cell, were contained within the lysosome that were present towards the center of the cell. After observing this phenomenon, they called it autolysis after the Nobel Prize winning Belgian cytologist and biochemist Christian de Duve and American Biologist Alex Benjamin Novikoff.

But, Porter and Ashford were wrong in interpreting their data and did not know that it was not autolysis, but rather a different process that they were observing. Later, in 1963, another group of biologists published a detailed descriptive study on "focal cytoplasmic degradation" (Hruban, 1963). In this study, these biologists found out that there were 3 stages which were happening continuously to sequester cytoplasm to lysosomes. After reading this, de Duve coined the phenomenon "autophagy," which he thought to be a part of lysosomal function. De Duve, along with his student, studied the phenomenon and came to the conclusion that lysosome was responsible for glucagon-induced autophagy. This was also the very first time that it was established that lysosomes are the sites where intracellular autophagy takes place. Some time later in the 1990s, autophagy related genes were discovered by several groups of scientists independently. These genes were discovered using the budding yeast process. Among these scientists was Yoshinori Ohsumi, who along with his partner Michael Thumm experimented with starvation induced non selective autophagy.

At the same time, another scientist named Daniel J. Klionsky also discovered another form of selective autophagy, which was the cytoplasm to vacuole targeting pathway (Klionsky, 1992). After a while, it was understood that everyone was looking at the same phenomenon from different perspectives. So, in 2003, a unified nomenclature was established, which was ATG, to refer to all the autophagy genes. Although different researchers were involved in the discovery of ATG, in 2016 Yoshinori Oshumi was awarded the Nobel Prize in Physiology or Medicine for this discovery.

The 21st century is when the field of autophagy really expanded and its growth was accelerated. The discovery of ATG helped scientists better understand the functions of autophagy, so much so that they were able to research the function of autophagy in diseases. A milestone discovery was made in 1999 which connected autophagy to cancer. This discovery was published by Beth Levine's group (Lahiri, 2018). Even at present, the main theme behind autophagy research is the relationship between cancer and autophagy. Another noteworthy event related to autophagy happened in 2003, when the first Gordon research Conference on autophagy was held. Other important events, like the launch of Autophagy, a scientific journal dedicated to this field in 2005, and the creation of BMHT fusion protein in 2008, also took place.

Uses of Autophagy

As already discussed, the main use of autophagy is to degrade or break down damaged organelles in cells or unused proteins. This also leads to the cells being repaired, and thus autophagy also acts as part of the repair mechanism. But aside from this, autophagy also has other important functions, too.

One of these is playing a role in various cellular functions. For example, in yeast, where high levels of autophagy are induced through nutrient starvation, besides degrading unnecessary proteins it also helps to recycle amino acids, which in turn are used to synthesize proteins that are important for survival. Nutrient depletion occurs in animals right after birth because of the severing of trans-placental food supply. This is also when autophagy comes into play, which helps to mediate this nutrient depletion.

Another one of the functions of autophagy is called xenophagy. Xenophagy is the breakdown of infectious particles through autophagy. Thus, autophagy also acts as a part of the immune system.

Chapter 2:

Autophagy: How it Works

We're about to get a little more technical in exploring the mechanics behind autophagy. It might get a little dense, so feel free to skip ahead if the science behind it doesn't interest you.

So, as you know by now, autophagy essentially recycles bits of your cells, and it does so in a few basic (the term "basic" is used here loosely) steps. The terms you need to know when it comes to autophagy are:

- vesicle: fluid filled sac in the body
- cytoplasm: the material in a cell
- phagophore: precursor to a vesicle, it encloses the cytoplasm during macroautophagy
- autophagosome: what the phagophore becomes, it plays the intermediary between cytoplasm and lysosome
- lysosome: waste removal organelle
- organelle: a specialized structure inside a cell

There will be other terms that might be unfamiliar, but these are the essential pieces that go into the process.

Essential Steps

There are 5 basic steps that take place through autophagy.

1. The phagophore is created by a protein kinase complex and a lipid kinase complex that work together to source a membrane that will become the phagophore.

2. Next comes phagophore expansion. In this stage, a particular protein known as LC3 is bonded with the newly formed phagophore through multiple autophagy-related proteins commonly known as ATG. After bonding with the phagophore, the LC3 protein becomes LC3-II. The formation occurs around the cytoplasm material that is to be degraded. This material can either be random, or it can be specifically selected if it includes damaged organelles and proteins that have been misfolded. When the replacement process starts occurring, a transmembrane protein called ATG-9 acts as the protector of the phagophore formation site and is commonly thought to help in expanding it by increasing the number of phagophore membranes by supplying them from nearby membrane locations.

3. The phagophore changes shape to become elongated and closes itself up, at which point it becomes an autophagosome. This autophagosome holds in the materials that will be degraded in a coming step.

4. Here's where the lysosome comes in. The autophagosome and the lysosome membranes fuse together. Within the lysosomal lumen (space within a lysosome), there are hydrolases. Hydrolases divide molecules into smaller pieces by using water to demolish chemical bonds. When the autophagosome and lysosome fuse together, the material inside the autophagosome is exposed to these chemical wrecking balls. This fusion also turns the lysosome into an autolysosome.

5. The hydrolases do their work and degrade the material within the autophagosome along with the inner membrane. The macromolecules that are created through this process are then shuffled around by permeases that are on the autolysosome

membrane until they're back in the original cytoplasm. The macromolecules can now be reused by the cell.

And that's how autophagy works! There are a few details we skipped over and terms that weren't explained, some of which will be explored below. If that made your head spin, though, don't worry! This is a complex biological science that is still being studied to further our understanding, so don't feel bad if it's over your head. It's still over a lot of heads!

Kinase

One term we skipped over was kinase, so we'll dedicate a short section to discussing what these are since they play an important role in autophagy.

Kinase, an enzyme which is present in cells, is responsible for the regulation of autophagy. When a variation of kinase called mTOR (mammalian target of rapamycin) is triggered, autophagy doesn't occur. The lack of it triggers autophagy in cells.

The lack of mTOR occurs when the body suffers from a lack of nutrition. The process is bound with the aggression and regression of glucagon and insulin. To understand their function in how autophagy works, let's give you a short rundown of them first. Glucagon, which is a peptide hormone, is created by alpha cells in our pancreas. Glucagon is considered vital for our bodily functions due to the fact that it is the main catabolic hormone (these are hormones responsible for maintaining and regulating the metabolic processes) of the human body responsible for important functions such as maintaining the regulation of glucose and fatty acids in the bloodstream.

Insulin is produced in the same pancreatic area of our body, except unlike glucagon, which is created by alpha cells, insulin is created by beta cells and is functionally the complete opposite of glucagon. It is the main anabolic hormone of the human body and mainly regulates the metabolic rate of carbohydrates and fat in the human body. The process of growth, regeneration, and degeneration of the cells of any living organism, including humans, is known as metabolism.

These two peptide hormones constantly play a tug-of-war wherein if the ratio of one goes up, the other goes down. Insulin goes down when the human body is starved of nutrition, which results in the increase of glycogen.

Autophagy is occurring in cells all the time passively at a base level to constantly make minor replacements and repairs to our body cells on a regular basis, but actively inducing it externally by nutrition is what kicks in the real benefits in the autophagy process. Intracellular molecules are digested when nutrition and oxygen starvation occur in cells, leading to digestion of said molecules by the cell as a replacement for nutrient instead.

Due to the sensitive balance that needs to be maintained for a healthy metabolic process of the body, autophagy needs to be greatly regulated and controlled to get the maximum benefit out of the process. Maintaining the amino acid levels in the body's cellular structure is mainly how this is done. Though there is no concrete evidence, many experts assume that signals are provided to the mTOR pathway automatically by cells when it receives certain signals from the cells indicating a lack of them. Once the amino acids enter the autophagy process, they are transferred to the liver for one of any three of the following functions: to be broken down into glucose via TCA (tricarboxylic acid), be part of the gluconeogenesis process, or recreated as new cellular protein. By performing these functions, the amino acid deposits in our body cells that would have been harmful in the long run are used up in a beneficial manner.

This is a relatively simple understanding of autophagy in mildly scientific terms. If you want to know further details of the process of autophagy, there are specialized books dedicated to how the autophagy process works that will give you a far more in depth view. In the next several chapters, the focus of this book will be on discussing the different benefits of autophagy, how to successfully activate and maintain it based on common body type classifications and nutrition recommendations, as well as its correlation with weight loss.

Chapter 3:

Benefits of Autophagy

To understand the benefits of autophagy, you need to have a basic understanding of how autophagy works in the context of health and its role in preventing different types of diseases.

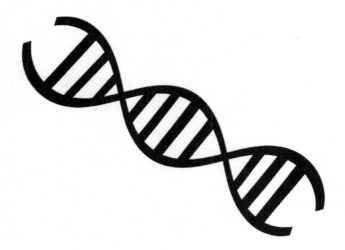

Many doctors and health experts consider autophagy as a double edged sword - it is useful under particular circumstances for some major brain degenerative disease as well as cancer, muscular disorders, liver diseases, and pathogen infections. It has its cons as well, unless it's done in a controlled fashion along with other accompanying treatments or processes. Some of the common benefits of autophagy in different types of major diseases include the following:

- Destruction of toxic protein cells.
- Residual protein recycling in diseased cells.
- Promoting cellular regeneration.

To cut a long story short, the degeneration of older cells and the creation of new cells are the main health benefits that autophagy brings to the table, along with other ones as well. By the cellular degeneration-regeneration process caused by autophagy, the anti-aging factors of the body get activated, keeping us looking and feeling younger.

The Benefits

Here are some of the major benefits that the knowledge and application of autophagy will bring into your life.

Improved Quality of Life

While there are a ton of techniques and methods out there guaranteeing health improvements and benefits, no amount of dieting or anti-aging creams will improve and benefit your health as much as autophagy. The cellular regeneration and degeneration processes caused by autophagy make you appear more youthful than your actual age. This is particularly important for our skin, which is constantly exposed to pollution, dust particles, and other things surrounding our lives which cause wrinkles and decrease skin quality by forming layers of toxic materials on skin cells.

Improvement in Body Metabolism

Autophagy is highly useful and productive as a metabolism booster. It does this by replacing and regenerating important metabolism related cells such as mitochondria. The digestive system of our body is also improved via autophagy, contributing to good body metabolism. This in turn affects the body's muscle performance by promoting cell growth and development of muscle mass in the correct areas of the muscles, preventing any kind of stress related muscle injuries. And despite the fluctuation of nutrition intake, the body can maintain its required weight through the improved metabolism induced by autophagy.

Improvement of the Body's Immune System

Autophagy is highly effective in keeping our body's immune system in tiptop shape. It does so in two ways: by promoting inflammation in cells and by actively fighting diseases via non-selective autophagy. Cellular inflammation boosts the immune system of cells when attacked by different types of diseases, and autophagy induces this inflammation by forcing the cell proteins to work more actively by starving them of nutrition. This in turn instigates the required immune response to keep infections and diseases at bay or eliminate harmful elements like microbacterium, tuberculosis, and other viral elements altogether from the cell itself.

Increased Cellular Lipid Homeostasis

As previously mentioned, autophagy and protease are linked with one another. This serves as the basis for the biological study on lipid mechanism. Recent studies into this subject matter have revealed that both of these major proteolytic degradative pathways are interlinked and directly influence lipid homeostasis. They're interlinked by the REGγ-SirT1 complex and perform different functions in cells depending on their protein composition. This has opened up possibilities to alternative treatment for different major metabolic disorders such as diabetes and liver osteosis.

Increased Cyclin A2 Degradation

In cell cycles, the degradation of a cellular component known as cyclin A2 is a vital part of the process. Autophagy has been proven to boost and regulate the process in recent studies.

Decreases Risk of Cancer

One of the biggest reasons autophagy has received such widespread attention among medical professionals and the general population alike is due to its preventive capabilities regarding cancer. Cancer is the result of particular cellular disorders, to put it in a nutshell, and autophagy actively helps in preventing these disorders by promoting cellular inflammation, regulating damage response caused to the DNA by different foreign bodies, and regulate genome instability.

Decreases Risk of Neurodegenerative Diseases

The risk of neurodegenerative diseases such as Parkinson's and Alzheimers can be significantly decreased through autophagy. Neurodegenerative diseases work on the basis of the accumulation of old and toxic neurons that pile up in particular areas of the brain and spread in surrounding areas. Autophagy replaces useless neuron parts and regenerates new ones, keeping these kinds of diseases in check.

Decreases Risk of Apoptosis (cell death)

When the cells of our body degrade beyond the point where they cannot be regenerated or replaced, cell death occurs, which is known as apoptosis in medical terminology. Apoptosis is bad, because the cells which are lost through cell death are irreparable, meaning that losing them once is losing them for a lifetime. Autophagy helps prevent this by a huge margin. Many deadly diseases are linked with cell death, so preventing it from the get-go is the best way to prevent those diseases, especially neurodegenerative ones.

Decreases Loss of Pigment Epithelial Cells

RPECs (Retinal Epithelial Cells) play a crucial role in the development of retinal cells responsible for our eyesight. Since our eyes are exposed to all kinds of foreign agents due to their open nature, this exposes their internal components without the protection of skin, resulting in endogenous and exogenous oxidative injuries. As a result, retinal cells suffer from constant damage more compared to other organ cells in the body. Though retinal cells have their own form of protection against the elements, autophagy provides a significant boost in maintaining and regulating RPEC functions.

Improves Digestive Health

The cells of your gastrointestinal tract are always working. Those cells work so much that part of them gets passed out as excreta. With autophagy, however, you get to repair your digestive cells, which can help get rid of junk. This will also activate the immune system appropriately.

Since a chronic gut immune response can inflame your bowels, it is important for them to constantly rest and get a chance to repair and restore. With autophagy and an extended night fast, you can give your gut the needed chance to relax and recharge.

Improves Your Skin

The skin, the largest organ in the body, is most susceptible to damage from sunshine, heat, adverse weather, air pollution, light, chemicals, changes in humidity, and other forms of damage. It is because of excessive damage that skin cells age faster. With autophagy, however, you not only replace new cells but also repair old ones so that it glows with health.

Skin cells help get rid of bacteria that infiltrate the body, hence you have to energize them so they are active with this protective assignment.

Regulates Inflammation

With autophagy, you can boost or reduce the immune response, whichever is needed, by promoting or preventing inflammation. In the presence of a dangerous invader, autophagy boosts inflammation by springing the immune system to attack.

Autophagy will, however, decrease inflammation in the immune system by getting rid of the signals causing it.

Helps Combat Infectious Disease

As discussed above, autophagy can help spring the immune system into action when needed. Also, with autophagy, you can get rid of some microbes from the body cells like Mycobacterium tuberculosis, or even deadly viruses such as HIV. Toxins that come about as a result of these infections can also be taken care of through the process of autophagy.

Overall Length of Life

The concept of autophagy is not new. As far back as 1950, scientists had discovered the process of autophagy and the tremendous potential it holds. Through it, you do not need to take in new nutrients, rather, encourage the process of autophagy through the recycling of damaged cell parts, getting rid of toxic body cells.

This process energizes the cells and renews their vigor. Anti-aging benefits might seem like a fallacy, but real beauty runs far deeper than the skin.

The Negative Side Effects of Autophagy

As enticing as the benefits of autophagy are, it does come with some side effects. Although these will be discussed in detail in a later part of the book, we thought to shed light on some of them.

Autophagy helps regulate inflammation and immunity by getting rid of inflammasome activators. Xenophagy is the process in which the body gets rid of pathogens via autophagy, which is beneficial to the immune system. Some bacteria, however, like coxiella, bartonella, and Brucella, will divide and multiply through autophagy. In other words, there is overgrowth of the bacteria.

ATG6/BECN1 is an autophagy gene that encodes the Beclin1 protein. It helps suppress tumors in cancer cells. Recently, however, it was discovered that its suppressing effect on cancer cells is not that impactful. In fact, its self replicating effect can even promote cancer cells. The process of self eating can make tumor cells resilient and survive against environmental stressors which make them survive chemotherapy and starvation. Hence, for cancer cells, autophagy is good as a preventive measure, rather than a treatment plan.

Research has yet to establish whether autophagy promotes apoptosis or programmed cell death. The result is a factor of the stimuli or cell types.

Malignant tumor cell as well, when they are subjected to nutritional stress via calorie deprivation, are preserved by autophagy by guarding against apoptosis.

Hence, with autophagy, it is not all black and white. While some pathogens, bacteria, and viruses will be destroyed by the process, others will use the process to thrive well. Also, autophagy reacts differently depending on the environment and surrounding tissues, for instance muscle, fat, brain, liver etc., which could be good or bad.

Chapter 4:

Macro and Micro Autophagy

In the first chapter, a brief outline was provided on the basics of macro and micro autophagy. In this chapter, we will go into more in depth into the details of these two autophagy types to understand how they influence our body and their benefits.

Macroautophagy

Macroautophagy is the process through which non-functional cellular constituents are catalyzed to the lysosome of the cells. What macroautophagy essentially does is separate the cytoplasm of cells, including different cell organs, and degrade them into amino acids. In Chapter 2, we had already discussed what mTOR is. In this chapter, we will go more into the term and its variations for the sake of explaining the functions of macroautophagy and how it works.

mTOR

mTOR has a complex known as mTORC1 (mTOR Complex-1) which is comprised of four main regulators: mLST8, PRAS40, RAPTOR, and DEPTOR. The first one is a positive receptor, while the second, third, and fourth ones are negative receptors. When cells starve from amino acids, mTORC1 deactivates in cytoplasm of cells while reactivating when amino acid levels become normal again. When mTORC1 is activated via amino acid simulation and enters the lysosomes, it promotes cell growth as well as protein synthesis. This process happens when a cellular constituent called RAG GTP activates upon amino acid simulation.

The primary link between the nutritional condition of cell and macroautophagy is a protein kinase or its replacement, Ulk1 and Ulk2. Fusing with Atg13 and FIP200, Ulk1 develops a complex formation that bolsters its activity and size. Ulk1/2 basically acts as the signal receptors of the macroautophagy process, letting the cell know when it is being starved.

The Stages of Macroautophagy

In the different stages of macroautophagy, the process differs a lot from microautophagy. In the first stage of macroautophagy, the process starts with the development of omegasomes in the cell which are developed by several macroautophagy inducing proteins and lipids in the ER (endoplasmic reticulum) membrane of cells. This omegasome then develops into phagophores, which essentially triggers the start of the autophagy process. Macroautophagy is categorized into 5 main categories: mitophagy, ribophagy, zymophagy, pexophagy, and lipophagy.

Macroautophagy caught attention in 1999 when a breakthrough was discovered, drawing a correlation between macroautophagy and cancer. The conflicting nature it plays in the disease still has scientists baffled. But, it is apparent that cellular senescence has something to do with it all. Macroautophagy plays a huge role in cellular senescence, which is the stationary status of a cell cycle. Cellular senescence is influenced by a couple of factors including genotoxic stress, inflammatory cytokines, and mitogens. The biggest importance of cellular senescence in modern day medical science is the role it plays in stopping the propagation of dead or damaged cells in surrounding areas. This process is externally induced during cancer treatment, the discovery of which was the key point of the breakthrough in autophagy in the 90s. After years of research by medical experts and scientists all around the globe, cellular senescence is now established as the aging process of cells.

So how does macroautophagy fit into all this? By influencing cellular senescence in multiple ways. The research into the relationship between macroautophagy and cellular senescence was done by Bergamini et al, whose research data and conclusion included a solid link between events occurring in cellular senescence and macroautophagy (Bergamini, 2007). Macroautophagy has a direct hand in the oncogene-induced senescence process in which it plays its part by degrading polyubiquitinated proteins, which are generated by the switch in proteasome to autophagy process through the increase of Bag3/Bag1 ratio in the oncogene-induced senescence process.

While macroautophagy is part of the transition process, its role as a direct influencer wasn't confirmed until the research findings of Young et al. The group of researchers led by Young found that the increase in macroautophagy levels were induced by the HrasV12 retroviral transduction during the senescence process via IMR90 cells which was not observed in cells that were still in a regenerative state, also known as quiescent cells (Young, 2009). This is paradoxical in nature, since autophagic activity and activation of mTOR in cells were occurring at the same time. This left researchers really baffled for a while.

A separate group of researchers led by Narita et al figured out the method behind the madness of this cellular paradox and published the results in their research journal which explained the phenomenon. According to their findings, the process that allowed both instances to be running within a cell at the same time was TASCC (TOR-autophagy spatial coupling compartment) (Narita, 2011). According to this concept, the cell actively hides mTOR activity from the macroautophagy elements present in the cell, effectively masking it so that neither interfere with the other's functions being carried out within the cell. By doing this, the target cell achieves high-level protein synthesis capabilities it would otherwise not have. This helps multiple vital organs like the kidneys to stay functional and effective.

Macroautophagy affects cells under different conditions. In normal cells, macroautophagy increases attenuation for senescence prematurely via glycated collagen I when HUVEC cell exposure is induced. Under this theory, lysosomal membrane permeabilization induces macroautophagy as a cellular stress response, leading to an occurrence known as senescence phenotype. This ensures autolysosome formation, which has been previously discussed, doesn't occur in an imbalanced manner so that transference to lysosomes becomes problematic later on.

When it comes to cells transformed by HrasV12 transduction, macroautophagy is accelerated and behaves in a different manner. This kind of macroautophagy is termed as RAS-activated autophagy, which is induced when there is deprivation of Atg5 or Atg7 constituents in the macroautophagy process of the transformed cell. When enough Atg5 is present, the RAS induced autophagy doesn't occur. Both Atg5 and Atg7 are molecular components which are thought to have different effects on macroautophagic fine-tuning. These findings clearly indicate that macroautophagy is deeply involved in cellular senescence.

Immortal Cells

The effect of macroautophagy on immortal cells, otherwise known as HeLa cells, supports the common research theory noted by many autophagy researchers that oncogene-induced senescence is directly influenced by macroautophagy. HeLa cells are not truly immortal - they are referred to as such because they are a particular cell-line that ignores and bypasses the effects of cellular senescence and keep continuing cell division. Due to this, immortal cells serve as the baseline for different branches of biological studies and research like biochemistry, biotechnology, and cell biology. According to Young et al's research documentation, in the case of immortal cells, the presence of a molecular element known as E1A, which is an adenoviral oncoprotein, suppresses RAS induced macroautophagic senescence (Young, 2009). Macroautophagy in immortal cells is also similarly dependant on Atg7-like transformed cells.

Chemo-Resistant Cells

Researchers have stumbled across some interesting results when it comes to studying autophagy in tumor tissue chemo-resistant cells. In these kinds of cells, senescence is triggered when long-term mTOR inhibition occurs. While this has occurred in particular research models, the exact opposite has also occurred in other research models pertaining to chemoresistant cells and autophagy, making it difficult to reach any solid conclusions.

When cell senescence is activated, SASP (senescence-associated secretory phenotype) is secreted as a result, which is a mixture of molecules and proteins that is a rich source of energy for the cells. SASP is mainly composed of tissue enzymes, cytokines, and chemokines. SASP mainly regulates and reinforces senescence phenotypes in cells which is a critical function in cell biology. Even though it is a rich energy source, SASP also comes with some particular drawbacks. These include inflammation during cleanup of senescence cells as well as the chance of increasing malignancy in cells.

Microautophagy

Now that we have the basics of macroautophagy out of the way, it is time for you to have a clear and concise idea about the second type of autophagy pathway known as microautophagy. Unlike macroautophagy, which focuses on cell cleanup, microautophagy thrives on the concept of dealing will cell survival under extreme external and internally induced conditions of the body. As such, it mainly regulates the size of cells, cellular starvation under nitrogen deprivation, as well as membrane homeostasis. Microautophagy works in tandem with macroautophagy for nutrient recycling when the body is starved willingly or unwillingly. Thus, this type of autophagy is non-selective in nature. The main difference between macroautophagy and microautophagy is the involvement of invagination and vesicle scission.

Chapter 5:

Activating Autophagy through Exercise, Ketosis, Fasting, and Intermittent Water Fasting

Fasting is the most popular autophagy practice in the world, followed by ketosis. In this chapter, we will detail how to use these popular techniques to promote autophagy in your body and keep your body at peak condition through cellular conditioning.

Exercise

Exercise is a very effective way to boost autophagy if you know how to do the right ones. Exercises bring multiple health benefits to the table, all of them useful in the long run. For starters, brain and peripheral tissues start stimulating autophagy faster when we work out, since the glucose uptake of the cells increases with the body in full motion. Damaged mitochondria in the heart and brain cells are also cleaned out faster through both cardio and aerobics exercises. For proper cellular homeostasis, a protein kinase called AMPK (5' AMP-activated protein kinase) is essential to be developed in a cell which is also more easily achievable through exercising.

As of now, aerobics physical training is the best way to induce autophagic stimulation in your body, while high altitude training has also proven to be very effective in inducing autophagy. Exercises for inducing autophagy in the body are done best when fasting and your body cells are already stressed out due to nutritional starvation. This is why aerobics or low intensity-cardio exercises are best for promoting autophagy - they stress the cells enough to boost the process without wearing them down. Since the intensity levels of these kinds of exercises are lower, cells get enough time to replenish energy from body fat stored within them to provide the required energy to our body without getting stressed. These exercises also affect the major muscle groups of the body. Sure, you won't be getting buffed like a body-builder lifting weights, but that is not the point; you will notice that your muscles have more energy to start performing heavier exercises without fear of injury. The reason for this is that the catabolic stressors of cells are enhanced by autophagy, increasing the body's capability for resistance training.

Common aerobic exercises include running, cycling, swimming, skiing, as well as martial arts like kickboxing and boxing. Other than promoting the processes of autophagy, these exercises also provide added protection to some of the most vital organs of the body like the heart and liver, along with aiding autophagic cellular repair. One of the key components of aerobics exercises is breathing, so mastering the art of breathing properly is also essential for doing aerobic exercises, which can be learned through meditation.

Ketogenic Diet

Now that we understand what autophagy truly is and are familiar with its function, it is quite clear that autophagy is a very important process that occurs in our body. But although autophagy is a natural process, it can be artificially boosted to get the most out of it. The literal meaning of autophagy is self-eating, and thus it is no surprise that fasting and dieting help to trigger autophagy.

The ketogenic diet is one of the main reasons why public attention has been drawn to the correlation between autophagy and dieting as a means for losing weight in a combined manner. The ketogenic diet is the most scientific diet that has been proven to actively promote autophagy and weight loss. The principal behind the ketogenic diet is reducing calorie intake without reducing the amount of food you are eating. A ketogenic diet promotes your cells to consume at least 75% of the required body calories from the fat stored in body cells, with the rest of the calorie intake to be obtained from carbohydrates. The ideal calorie intake percentage from carbohydrates in ketogenic diet is 10%. Through a ketogenic diet, the effects of fasting are stimulated within the human body without actually starving throughout the day. This is done by inducing ketogenesis, the process that forces cells to consume fat in the absence of enough glucose in the body.

There are several types of ketogenic diets, with the most prominent ones being the following:

- SKD (Standard Ketogenic Diet)
- CKD (Cyclical ketogenic Diet)
- TKD (Targeted Ketogenic Diet)
- HKD (High-protein ketogenic diet)

All of the above mentioned diets have some major differences which affect body types differently, hence the necessity of their differentiation. The standard ketogenic diet is low on carbs and high on fat. The nutrient distribution ration for it is 75% fat, 20% protein and 5% carbs. HKD is almost similar but richer in protein content as far as the nutrition content goes. The cyclical diet is a lot like crossfit exercising - a fusion of low and high intensity carbohydrate intake on alternating days. TKD is a keto diet that is based around workouts and exercises.

Ketogenic Foods and Drinks

Some of the common foods and beverages that can help induce autophagy in your body that are acceptable on a ketogenic diet are ginger, ginger tea, green tea, coffee, coconut oil, as well as reishi mushroom. While coffee can be immensely helpful, too much of it isn't good, so avoid having more than a cup or two when maintaining a ketogenic diet. Ginger has immense health benefits including destroying lung cancer cells. It also contains 6-shogaol, an active component that promotes autophagy. Coconut oil is the most effective, however, as it tricks the body into starving due to being plentiful in ketones, the same ones that are produced in our bodies.

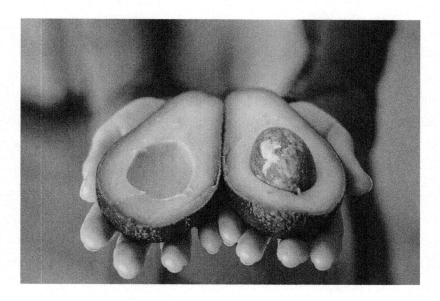

Like coconut oil, seafood is also highly ketogenic, so it makes the top of the list for maintaining a ketogenic diet. Vegetables are a definite no-brainer - just stick to vegetables that are low-carb. Most low-carb vegetables are high in minerals. Cheese and avocado are both delicious and healthy foods which are keto-friendly, but unfortunately both tend to be on the expensive side when it comes to price. Meat, poultry, and dairy consumption should be done in limited amounts. If you're a fruit aficionado, then go full squirrel-mode and stock up on various types of nuts and berries like raspberry, blueberry, and strawberry. There is also a strict outline of the types of food you should avoid. Sugary food or anything that has a high carbohydrate content for that matter needs to be avoided at all costs. Overly sugary fruits and root vegetables, especially potatoes, should be avoided on a ketogenic diet. Alternate between fruit, meats, and vegetables in your meals everyday and you will find that the ketogenic diet is easy enough to adapt to with the right mindset and restrictions. But, the most effective food item on this list would be fish.

Ketogenic Benefits

The benefits of a ketogenic diet aren't limited to weight loss only. It also has a host of other benefits, as well. It is highly beneficial in cancer and heart disease prevention, acne prevention, epilepsy, and neurodegenerative disorders. But a ketogenic diet also has its drawbacks - first of all there is the keto flu, which is the body's withdrawal symptoms to the nutritional imbalance caused at the beginning of a ketogenic diet. Then there's the fact that to supplement calorie intake, protein based meals lead to higher fat intake which can be very risky for the heart after a certain age threshold if a healthy lifestyle is not maintained. In extreme cases, a ketogenic diet can even cause nutritional deficiencies.

Intermittent Fasting

What makes intermittent fasting different? For starters, intermittent fasting occurs when a certain eating pattern is followed. This eating pattern involves a cycle between periods of eating and periods of fasting. This type of fasting is not concerned with which types of foods you eat. Rather, this specifies when you eat them. The most common intermittent fasting methods involve fasts that last up to 16 hours daily, or fasting for 24 hours two times a week. Fasting is actually a common practice that people from different religious backgrounds take part in, including Muslims, Christians, Judaist, etc. Intermittent fasting is just a modified version of this ancient practice.

There are quite a few different types of intermittent fasting. Although different in process, all of these have a common underlying theme, which is splitting the day or week into eating and fasting periods. Also, during the fasting periods of all of these methods, one is to eat very little to no food.

The most popular methods among the different intermittent fasting methods are:

The 16/8 Method

This is among the most common fasting methods and is also discussed briefly above. In this method, an 8-hour period is picked for eating and the remaining 16 hours are used for fasting. This method of intermittent fasting is also called the leangains protocol. You may also hear it referred to as the 8-hour eating window fast. It is one of the easiest forms of intermittent fasting, as it only requires you to skip breakfast or dinner and eat the other two meals of the day as you normally would.

Eat-Stop-Eat

This is the second method that was discussed earlier briefly. This method involves fasting for a whole day, that is 24 hours, once or twice a week. For example, you eat dinner at 9pm today and fast the whole day tomorrow until 9pm.

The 5:2 Fast

This method is closer to dieting, since here you eat normally 5 days a week and eat only 500-600 calories on the remaining two days. For this type of fast, you might decide to fast on Mondays and Wednesdays (consuming just 500 calories), while you take your normal meals for the remaining days.

Crescendo

This is a type of intermittent fasting that will not disturb your hormonal balance. With this type of fast, you take a couple of days to stay away from food for a maximum period of 16 hours. For instance, you could go without food for about 13 hours on Mondays, Wednesdays, and Fridays, and eat normally for the remaining days. It is a safe form of intermittent fasting, as the fasting window falls between 12 to 16 hours while the eating window is within the range of 8 to 12 hours.

20:4 Fast

As you can deduce from the name, your eating window all happens within 4 hours. For instance, you might eat all your meals in a day between 12 pm and 4 pm and avoid food for the next 20 hours. Between the four hour windows you have, you could eat one or two meals. However, be sure you do not binge eat, and always make the meals nutritious. This type of intermittent fast is best done twice or three times a week.

Extended Fasting

This is the best type of fasting you should aim for if autophagy is your goal. The human body is well equipped to survive going without food for days, even up to a week or two. This is, however, best done under the supervision of a health practitioner. It should be noted that extended fasting could have negative effects on your health, hence it should be moderated.

One Meal a Day Fasting

Like the name, you are required to eat once and wait for a 24 hour period before your next meal. Thus, if your meal today ends by 3:45 pm, your next meal should start by 3:45 pm the next day. While OMAD allows you eat daily, you eat in a controlled amount. It is a safe fasting type that should be considered just once or twice a week.

All of these methods can actively help to reduce weight, since they restrict the amount of calories you take in. The simplest among these methods is the 16/8 method, since it is easier to follow. You can easily choose a 16 hour fasting window in which 8 hours can be spent sleeping.

Since fasting is the process where the intake of food is stopped, this also results in your body using the existing resources to fuel itself. This in turn initiates the autophagy process which also helps in cellular repair. In fact, autophagy is considered as one of the main advantages of intermittent fasting, among others.

Other changes that are induced due to intermittent fasting are:

Increased Human Growth Hormone(HGH): When you fast, the levels of different growth hormones in your body increase drastically.

They have been observed to have increased up to 5 times. This in turn accelerates fat loss and muscle gain.

Decreased Levels of Insulin: Through intermittent fasting, the levels of insulin in the body decreases by a lot. On the other hand, this also increases insulin sensitivity in the body. Insulin sensitive means how responsive to insulin your cells are. The decreased levels of insulin make stored body fat more accessible for different biological processes.

Better Brain Health: Another change that occurs when you take part in intermittent fasting is that the brain hormone BDNF increases in amount. It also helps in the growth of new nerve cells. Additionally, this type of fasting can help to protect against Alzheimer's disease.

Just like everything else, intermittent fasting is not perfect, since it also has side effects. The main side effect of this is obviously hunger, which may lead to low productivity and also nausea. Intermittent fasting is something that takes time to get used to. Although the side effects of fasting may not be severe, it can become dangerous for people with diabetes, low blood pressure, eating disorders, women who are pregnant, and even people who are on medication. Thus, it is advised that people with these conditions consult with their doctors before taking on intermittent fasting.

Even though fasting is good for human physiology, there are times when it is better not to fast than to fast. People with eating disorders or with anemia definitely shouldn't fast due to nutritional issues. Any kind of fasting should be avoided by pregnant women as well. People with diabetes and kidney disorders should refrain from fasting.

Another thing to keep in mind is how long you are fasting and how your body is adapting to it. If your body has quick adaptation mechanics, then fasting will lead to consumption of muscle protein instead of fat, which is bad for your body mass.

Intermittent Water Fasting

Intermittent water fasting is sensitive and strenuous for the human body, so it should only be done under proper supervision of physician or a nutritionist, as messing with your body's water mass is nothing to scoff at. Water fasting is basically total starvation of the human body with no liquid intake or solid food intake other than water. This makes it dangerous and sensitive in nature, as it leaves the body with no option to reinvigorate itself. This kind of fasting is usually done for 3 days for most normal folks, and some extend it up to 7-10 days.

Water fasting basically boils down to mental strength mostly, so start with one or two days of water fasting before trying out longer stretches.

Chapter 6:

Weight Loss and Autophagy

There are many, many health benefits of intermittent fasting. Among these are weight loss, autophagy, and overall healthy living. After many studies and extensive reading on intermittent fasting, I can confidently tell you that it is one of the best and most potent ways to lose excess fat.

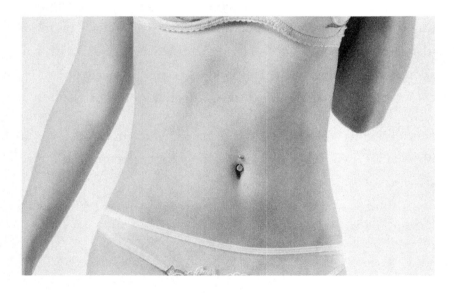

Think about it: you are depriving your body of energy, the energy it needs from the intake of food consistently. The body has no choice but to turn to stored fat as a source of energy. With time, if the fast is consistent, this leads to considerable weight loss.

It should be noted here that fat loss differs from weight loss. Besides, the fact that you are losing fat does not definitely translate to healthy living or activating autophagy. In actual fact, conventional diets that restrict calories might not get you to trigger autophagy.

Bear in mind that the healthy aging and longevity benefits that you get from fasting come up as a result of autophagy. This is why someone who doesn't aid their body in inducing autophagy will easily grow old and fall susceptible to disease.

The Concept of Lipolysis and Lipophagy

Lipolysis is a process in which body fats gets released from adipose stores. This fosters the shedding of body fat. Lipophagy, on the other hand, is a process in which autophagy helps with the breakdown of triglycerides, fatty acids, and cholesterol.

Lipophagy employs 'acid' lipolysis to break down cellular triacylglycerols in lysosomes that store fatty acids. Lipophagy metabolizes lipid stores which aids in fuelling mitochondrial beta-oxidation for it to maintain energy equilibrium. When lipophagy is disturbed, it encourages fatty livers.

The volume of lipid that gets broken down via the lipophagy process depends on how extracellular nutrient gets supplied to the body as well as the body calorie level. The nutritional status determines the amount of cell lipophagy.

Does Autophagy Help You Lose Fat?

The percentage of fat mass that a person has is determined by the number of adipocytes. However, it is said that the number of fat cells one has does not change even when the person loses weight. Every year, an adult renews about 10% of their fat cells.

41

Autophagy as a process that increases the rate of cell renewal. You, however, might not lose fat with autophagy unless you are really deficient in calories. For instance, staying away from food for 3 days and overeating will not help lose weight, even if you got to the point where autophagy started.

With the above in mind, autophagy is not directly related to fat loss, as it is determined by the overall energy balance of the body. Autophagy, however, promotes the breakdown of lipids and fatty acids with the process of ketosis and lipophagy.

Chapter 7:

Misconceptions and Lies about Autophagy

Over the years, the concept of intermittent fasting has gained wide acceptance. Since many people have seen the tremendous health benefits that come with fasting, the spotlight has been directed on it. With this increased focus on intermittent fasting and autophagy, many people have come up with speculations that are somewhat untrue about the concept.

Autophagy is a broad field with many new things to learn. I have dedicated this chapter to debunking the myths about the subject. As a recap, bear in mind the following:

- Autophagy is a catabolic state of the body that comes up as a result of reduced energy in the body. With reduced energy levels, AMPK is activated. AMPK is a fuel that supports autophagy.

- Reduced insulin level is also critical to the onset of autophagy. This is because autophagy encourages energy storage.

- Excess glucose in the body is also not good for autophagy because it triggers the release of insulin and reduces AMPK levels.

- Too much protein and amino acids in the body works against autophagy, as it raises the level of mTOR.

- There are many ways to promote autophagy. Exercise, fasting, and calorie restriction are some of the best known methods.

With the above in mind, the rest of this chapter will shed light on some false beliefs that many people have held onto about autophagy. Alongside this, we will debunk these ideas with proof and facts.

A 24 Hour Fast Can Help Trigger Autophagy

Even if you do get to trigger autophagy, you cannot get any significant boost with a 24 hour fast. If you want autophagy to start in such a short time, then a high-intensity exercise regimen is recommended. A 16 hour fast as well will not trigger any autophagy since it is a short time period. The following explains why:

Fasting does not happen right after finishing your last meal. As you know, the body will digest the ingested food nutrients and still draw energy from it.

After your last fast, the body remains in a postabsorptive state of metabolism for four hours.

Also, the fact that some food takes an extended period to digest adds to this time. Foods like vegetables, fibers, protein, and fat do not digest that easy.

As a result, the reality is that the body does not get into the fasted state until after 5 to 6 hours of going without food. This is because before that, you are still fed, and the body is thriving on the calories you consumed.

For instance, a person who took his last meal at 7 pm will not start the real physiological fast till around midnight. Thus, if you claim to be going on a 16 to 20 hour fast, the number of hours you have really spent fasting is only about 12 hours. This is way too short to trigger autophagy.

However, this does not mean there will not be other benefits of intermittent fasting. You could get reduced levels of insulin, low inflammation levels, and even fat burning.

More Autophagy is Better

Three days fast is the minimum time you need to experience significant autophagy. By the third day of your fast, you get to enjoy the benefits of fasting and autophagy, because this is when you energize your body to fight off tumors, cancer cells, and also boost stem cells production. I, however, need to submit here that more might not be the best.

In fact, there could be side effects with prolonged autophagy. Here are some of the adverse effects of protracted autophagy:

- Autophagy provides the perfect ground for some parasites such as Brucella and bacteria to reproduce.
- Tumor cells can develop tough skin which makes them strong and resilient. As a result of this, they become resistant to treatment.
- ATG6/BECN1, an essential autophagy gene that encodes the Beclin1 protein, is vital to reducing cancer cells. It could also feed cancer cells, however, giving them the needed strength to survive.
- There is a risk of sarcopenia and muscle wasting with excessive autophagy. This affects longevity.

Without a doubt, autophagy is incredible. We would not even be talking about it if it did not hold amazing health benefits. However, autophagy all the time isn't good for your body. You might trigger unwanted health repercussions and other health hazards that science has not yet shed light on.

The best approach to getting the best from autophagy is to induce it intermittently. You can have successive periods of fasting and feasting to enjoy autophagy. This is better than turning autophagy into a constant process.

Autophagy Equals Starvation

Some people also hold the belief that autophagy and intermittent fasting make you starve. This is far from the truth. Even though you have to stay away from food to accomplish autophagy, it is different from fasting.

If you want to get an idea of what starvation is, pictures kids from third world countries with protruding bones and bloated stomachs. That is a good illustration of starvation, and staying away from food for a couple of days will not make this happen to you. Besides, people starving rarely have the needed energy to go about their day to day activities, while someone who is practicing intermittent fasting still has energy.

While intermittent fasting, you will not deprive your body of the needed energy because:

- The body stores unused energy in the form of fats. It resorts to this energy in times of food scarcity. Even if you are very lean, with around just 10% body fat, this still translates to an average of 45,000 calories. This can keep you going for weeks.
- The process of autophagy breaks down old cells and protein in the body. This serves as an additional source of energy when you are not feeding. Hence, while fasting, the body will turn on other body components as a source of energy.
- After some days of fasting, you get to experience ketosis. In other words, the normal metabolism process is suspended since no new food intake is forthcoming. This transitions the body into ketosis, a process where the body uses stored fats and ketones as the energy that powers the brain and muscle. This makes you tap into another

46

abundant reservoir of fuel in the body, which can keep you going for days, even weeks.

- You get to improve your lifespan and longevity via basal autophagy. This is one of the keys to a long life that comes from restricting calories.

As indicated and explained above, the process of intermittent fasting and autophagy is way different from starvation. During fasting and autophagy, the body undergoes a process of healing and self-renewal, a process that does not take place in the feasting state — seeing it as starvation is just a wrong way of looking at it.

Autophagy Makes You Build Muscle

The process of building muscle requires calories. As a result of this, building muscle will be hard, if not near impossible, when there is no additional energy source and while staying away from food. Protein is also essential to build muscle, as it requires a vital process known as muscle protein synthesis.

With intermittent fasting, however, your protein intake is already limited. This switches the body to a catabolic state in which it breaks down, rather than the anabolism state where it grows.

It should be pointed out that the process of autophagy still can break down old protein molecules floating around your body cells. This can be a functional ingredient in muscle protein synthesis. The problem, however, is that some essential amino acids that are critical to muscle protein synthesis such as leucine will be absent.

This explains why it is pretty rare for someone overweight to start building muscle and lose body fats after commencing resistance training.

Autophagy Eats Up Your Loose Skin

There is a belief that autophagy can shrink your loose skin and tighten it up after you have lost weight. This is not entirely true. Some studies shed light on this.

In 2014, there was a study in Japan that established that aging fibroblast had reduced levels of autophagy (Kim, 2018). Fibroblast is responsible for skin collagen, which in turn is responsible for wrinkles and loose skin.

In Korea, there was a study in 2018 that revealed that aging fibroblast has a higher speed of waste, which makes the skin age (HS, 2018). According to the researchers, autophagy is critical to making people look younger by slowing down the aging process of the skin.

As established above, through autophagy, you can slow down the aging process which is revealed most prominently in the skin. However, autophagy does not consume loose skin and wrinkles. It does, however, foster the process that keeps the skin healthy and elastic, which makes it tighten faster.

Intermittent fasting, coupled with autophagy, can help guard against extreme loose skin when you lose a lot of weight. You might not be able to escape loose skin after shedding off a lot of body fat. The good news, however, is that if your weight loss comes from fasting, there will be increased levels of autophagy, which helps the skin fit perfectly to your new body fat.

If you subject yourself to restrictive calorie diets and lose weight without the process of autophagy, you will surely have loose skin. As indicated in the studies above, autophagy is the key to keeping the production of collagen and fibroblast active.

Fat Does Not Stop Autophagy

While fat will not spike your insulin levels the way proteins or carbs do, it does transition you to a fed state.

Ketosis fosters macroautophagy in the brain by enhancing Sirt1. With ketone bodies as well, chaperone-mediated autophagy gets activated in the organization which works on individual substrates and amino acids. While fasting in addition to being on the ketogenic diet, ketones and Beta-hydroxybutyrate levels increase.

mTor will not, however, respond to amino acid and glucose alone, but to all available calories. The summary here is that if there is excess energy, whatever the source, it will suppress autophagy.

While fat will not wholly stop autophagy, it will slow it down to a certain level. However, the amount of fat you have eaten will determine if fat prevents autophagy or not. Even a small amount, as small as a single tablespoon of MCT oil, will improve chaperone-mediated autophagy due to the increased levels of ketone bodies. Keep in mind that anything above 100 calories from fat will work against you.

BCAAs Do Not Stop Autophagy

Branched-Chain Amino Acids are composed of amino acids in its pure form. Even in trace amount, it will stop the autophagy process.

While fasting, you do not have to be afraid of losing muscle once you can maintain autophagy and stay in ketosis. As a result of the elevation of ketones, both will prevent the breakdown of muscle tissues.

Bear in mind, however, that if you do not get to stay in ketosis, and the autophagy process stops while fasting, you might lose muscle. This is confirmed when there is inadequate protein and other essential body nutrients. The main point you should note is that the consumption of BCAAs will result in the above as it translates you into the fed state, stopping ketosis.

You do not need high levels of BCAAs while fasting since the body is already burning glucose alongside an elevated level of blood sugar.

Eating Meat Will Not Make You Get Autophagy

Many people hold on to the fact that meats or other diets high in protein will work against autophagy, and you might age quickly.

In talking about autophagy, the frequency of eating is fundamental. If you do not fast more than 24 hours, and your three square meal is always complete, significant autophagy might be alien to you, even if you limit protein or meat consumption.

As established some chapters above, intermittent fasting coupled with calorie restriction is the best way to get autophagy on a carnivorous diet. Bear in mind, also, that insulin and carbs do not help autophagy. Hence, an entirely plant-based vegan diet will not help autophagy.

Eating Fruits Will Not break autophagy

Fruits do contain fructose which can be digested by the liver and stored as liver glycogen. Too much of this fructose is quickly converted into triglycerides.

Fruits work against autophagy and ketosis because it encourages the storage of liver glycogen. It is the content of glycogen in the liver that ensures the balance between the AMPK and mTOR. We can liken the liver to the central hub for energy metabolism and nutrients in the body.

Consuming fruits with a regulated amount of protein and fats could help you remain in the catabolic state of breaking down molecules. The chance of autophagy, however, is pretty slim. Autophagy is not the same as muscle loss and catabolism. Even in deep autophagy state, you can maintain your muscle mass. In the same way, you can be deep in ketosis, without autophagy and lose a significant amount of muscle mass.

The fruit is not the bad guy here. In specific amounts, it is healthy. However, you should rethink fruits if you want to maintain autophagy.

Coffee Hinders Autophagy

Coffee will neither break your fast nor work against autophagy. On the contrary, coffee is good for inducing ketosis and autophagy.

Coffee contains polyphenols, a compound that promotes autophagy. Coffee itself supports the process of autophagy through many other means. With caffeine also, the body enjoys lipolysis, which burns fat and reduces insulin, improves ketones and boosts AMPK.

Coffee will not hinder autophagy although; you will have to take it black, without cream, milk or sweeteners. This is because all of the above will increase insulin level and stop any benefit you will get from your fast. Dairy and milk, importantly, increases the level of IGF-1 which activates mTOR

You Cannot Have Autophagy While Eating

We do not dispute the fact that the surest way to activate autophagy is staying away from food. There are, however, some food items that can promote autophagy. While a chapter will be dedicated to this in the course of the book, some of the foods are:

- Tumeric and Curcumin boost autophagy
- Ginger triggers autophagy
- Cruciferous vegetable and Sulforaphane from broccoli enhances autophagy
- From red wine, dark berries and Skin of grapes, you get resveratrol which stimulates autophagy
- Medicinal mushroom also helps with autophagy

You will still need to restrict calorie consumption for you to get the full benefits of autophagy

Exercise Stops Autophagy

Exercise is one of the proven ways of boosting autophagy. In fact, in the brain and other peripheral tissues, activity triggers autophagy.

You can increase mTOR signaling via resistance training. While exercise will not turn on mTOR same way eating does, what exercise does is to translocate mTOR complex near the cellular membrane. It prepares it for action as soon as you start eating. When you work out, you become more sensitive to activating mTOR, which triggers more growth after the workout.

Also, you activate autophagy through in-depth resistance training, which could help reduce the destruction and breakdown of a muscle cell by regulating IGF-1 and its receptors.

Besides staying away from food, the best approach to increase autophagy is via workout. However, you get the best result when you combine both.

Final Thoughts

As it has been examined, there are some false believes that have been held about the concept of autophagy. But we hope that as you continue on the quest to reward yourself with this health process, you take note of the lies that might hinder your success.

Chapter 8:

Water Fasting and Autophagy

Water fasting, even though it is a fast, differs from intermittent fasting. This is because water fasting involves staying away from food and drinks entirely for a given period, the duration of the fast. In other words, you only drink water to suppress hunger throughout the fast. Water fasting can range from 24 hours to 72 hours, depending on what you want. It is, however, not recommended that you exceed 72 hours.

Worthy of note is the fact that people should be careful before starting a water fast. The advice of an expert, such as a dietician or doctor, is vital before attempting a water fast. People fast for many reasons. Two of the most important reasons are to shed off excess fat and detoxify the body (autophagy).

As indicated above, when you fast, you go without food for hours or days depending on what you want. The intention is to induce autophagy.

Pregnant women, people with chronic kidney issues, as well as people with a history of eating disorders should not try water fasting. This is because of the intensity of the fast and the limitations it places on individuals. We recommend a maximum of 72 hours due to the side effects that could arise from fasting. If you would like to extend the fast, the advice of a doctor is non-negotiable. Besides, you can consider retreat centers that offer fasting programs where you are under the constant supervision of health practitioners where you can be easily supported.

Worthy of note is the fact that you should not stress your body too much while trying water fasting because of the side effects associated with it. You might not be able to escape dizziness and lightheadedness on the fast, especially if you're a first timer.

All in all, make sure you avoid driving or operating heavy machinery while on a water fast. The next part explores the benefits and side effects of water fasting.

Water Fasting Pros

There are many reasons why people fast. It could be for religious or health reasons. If you are going to undergo a surgery in the hospital, for instance, you will have to stay away from food. This shows that there is something special about fasting and health. Fasting comes in many forms. Water fasting, unlike other types of fasting, is highly restrictive because you get zero calories and no food at all. You have to be determined and mentally prepared, as it is not going to come on a bed of roses. With that aside, many health benefits come with water fasting. This part of the book will shed light on these.

Cell Regeneration or Autophagy

Since the theme of this book is autophagy, I believe it is okay to start with autophagy as one of the health benefits of water fasting. Cellular regeneration is one of the main advantages of water fasting. Also known as autophagy, it is the natural ability of the body to get rid of dysfunctional cells. Water fasting forces the body to go into an induced state of autophagy. What happens is that the body will have to choose which cells are relevant and functioning, to keep them protected, and also ensure they get adequate nutrients, since nutrient intake is limited already.

At the same time, the body disposes of old cells that are no longer relevant in the body. It also creates new, durable, and healthy body cells as a replacement for the ones disposed of. The ability of the body to get rid of these damaged body cells and replace them with new, healthy ones improves the healing capacity of the body.

Slows Down Aging

You not only get to enjoy autophagy with water fasting. Many other tremendous health benefits come with water fasting, one of which is slowed down aging. When there is an excess supply of oxygen in the body, it triggers an abundance of free radicals, which results in cellular oxidation, which also causes premature aging.

When you go into water fasting, however, the body cells already damaged by free radicals get expelled. This makes way for new, young, and healthy body cells, which translates to looking and feeling young. Bear in mind that when you expel old body cells, you make the body stronger, with a renewed capacity to fight off disease, infections, and germs. Hence, it is more than just aesthetic as some may think. Besides, new body cells can communicate with each other better to keep the body healthy.

Weight Loss

Generally, it is expected that when you stay away from food for a given period, the body goes into ketosis. It is usually not until you eat the ketogenic diet that you get into ketosis. The body goes into ketosis because no more food is coming in; hence, it is forced to turn on its reserve – fats. It derives energy from fats stored in the body and breaks them down.

Thus dieting, as well as water fasting, can get you into ketosis, which leads to the burning of fat. You, however, need to know that ketosis makes the body draw needed energy from body fat. As a result of this, you have to be careful about the activities you do during water fasting due to the restricted calorie intake. Feeling lightheaded is common during water fasting partly thanks to ketosis.

Improved Insulin Receptivity

The pancreas creates a hormone called insulin, which helps keep the blood sugar level of the body in check. When you fast, the body gets better at controlling spikes in glucose levels. Not only that, but the body can also send these hormones to keep the blood sugar level from rising. Since the body becomes more sensitive to insulin, there is a lower risk of developing diabetes now or later in life.

Reduced Risk of Cancer and Heart Disease

There is evidence to support the fact that water fasting does help reduce the risk of cancer and heart disease. This is not surprising, as this benefit of water fasting is the offshoot of cell cleansing (autophagy) and reduced inflammation.

Also, there is evidence to support the fact that water fasting may slow or even completely stop the growth of tumors. Not only that, but it also improves the effectiveness of chemotherapy while helping to reduce the side effects. As a result, cancer treatment, when combined with water fasting, gives terrific results.

Also, as indicated above, water fasting helps get rid of free radicals in the body. This keeps the heart protected from any damage that might come from free radicals.

Reduced Blood Pressure

To reduce blood pressure, health practitioners advised limiting salt intake and increasing water intake. This is the basis of water fasting. Hence, it automatically helps manage and reduce blood pressure. Even people with hypertension can show significant improvement if they water fast under medical supervision.

Possible Side Effects of Water Fasting

As emphasized above, water fasting is highly restrictive. Hence, it does come with several side effects that you should note. This will help you decide if it is worth exploring or not. Also, it is essential I drive home the fact that the water fast is best and safer with the supervision of a medical practitioner. This is because they will be more equipped in helping to manage the associated side effects.

With the above in mind, expect and be prepared for the following when going on a water fast.

Dehydration

This is somewhat ironic, I must admit, but bear in mind that the possibility of getting dehydrated is high while on a water fast. This is because the body gets some percentage of its water in the food ingested; however, water fasting restricts you from any form of food at all.

This is why dehydration is possible with water fasting as well. As a result, an increased amount of water intake is essential during a water fast. Keep in mind that with dehydration, the chances of feeling lightheaded and dizzy also increase.

Unintended Weight (Muscle) Loss

It is the loss of fat in the body that translates to weight loss. Although fat also serves as energy reserves in the body, it has no other use in excess amounts. One bad thing about a water fast is that the body loses muscle weight, which is not good. This is because muscle is vital to keep the metabolism active even while resting, keeping the body from shock.

Muscle also helps as you go about your day to day activities. However, since the body has no access to calories while water fasting, you will not only lose shape fast, but lose muscle weight as well.

Heartburn and Stomach Ulcers

The intake of food to the stomach is paused. This causes the digestive system to go on a break. Stomach acid with no purpose can trigger stomach ulcers and heartburn. The possibility of this is high, especially if you have had it in the past.

However, adequate water intake is a way to help reduce the impact of stomach ulcers and heartburn.

There are other side effects, but these are the basics. Bear in mind that one of the easiest ways to induce autophagy is via water fasting. It even proves faster than exercise or other means. This is why we thought to explore water fasting in detail. If you would like to go on a water fast, the next section discusses how to get started and many other things to expect.

Getting Started With Water Fasting

The best and safest way to go about water fasting is with the help of a doctor. Their expertise is significant in guiding you on what to expect and also to mitigate the associated side effects. Also, should any health conditions arise as a result of the fast, you will be able to manage with ease.

When fasting, planning is vital. If you have never fasted before, it is not recommended to jump into three days of water fasting. That is not ideal. As effective as water fasting is, if done improperly, it could cause more harm than good. This is why you have to plan well.

What to Expect During a Water Fast

The period of water fasting is a time to rest, not stress your body in any form. Since there is no calorie intake coming in, you should strive to preserve the little energy reserve your body uses to survive. Therefore, this is not the time to go out partying or exercising strenuously - instead, you need to sleep. Your body needs it. Be sure to listen to the demands of your body and give in to more sleep to compensate for the deprived energy. Sleep during the day, and get 10 hours or more of sleep in the night. This is nothing out of the ordinary. Embrace and enjoy the process.

Be sure to concentrate on taking in at least 2 liters of water per day. Of course, you are not drinking all this at once. Instead, you drink it throughout the day to keep yourself hydrated.

Water fasting comes with many health benefits; however, it will not come on a platter of gold, as the first couple of days will be tough. There will be unpleasant symptoms such as irritability, disorientation, and extreme hunger. The good news, however, is that you have a healthy body that can adapt fast. By the third day, you should feel much better.

When on a water fast, it is essential you plan your schedule. We advise staying off work for the period of the fast. Or better still, schedule your fast for the weekend if time off will be impossible. Also, chose the fasting duration you want. As indicated earlier, water fasting should not last for too long. If you are a beginner, we recommend a day or a maximum of three days.

Concentrate More on High Quality Water

Fresh, clean, and high-quality water is the best to consume while on a water fast. Should the water you drink be laden with impurities, you will see the side effects quickly as the absence of food rapidly magnifies this. With the above in mind, be sure to concentrate only on distilled water while on your water fast. Filtered or boiled water is also a good idea.

It is important to reiterate that fasting is not for pregnant or lactating mothers. Nutritional deficiencies might hurt a developing child. Also, people with type 1 diabetes should not go for water fasting. People who are underweight as well should try other means to induce autophagy, rather than water fasting. If you have less than 20 pounds you want to lose and you want it to go fast, be sure you don't follow a protracted fast.

If you are determined and ready to go on with water fasting, make sure you proceed with caution and the right mindset.

Final Thoughts

We have introduced water fasting as one of the most efficient ways of inducing autophagy. Water fasting is an extreme form of fasting that comes with side effects, but tremendous health benefits. Water fasting will get you into autophagy faster than exercise and calorie restriction. However, water fasting needs to be regulated and controlled. Extended durations of fasting are best done under the supervision of a doctor.

The next chapter discusses the essential tips on getting started with water fasting.

Chapter 9:

Tips on Having a Smooth Water Fast

Water fasting, unlike intermittent fasting, is pretty extreme. It must be done with extreme caution and preparation. Since there is no intake of calories at all, it is pretty challenging. So, you have to be prepared to ensure your fast goes smoothly.

This chapter is all about guiding you with tips to go about water fasting to reap the tremendous health benefits, autophagy included. Make sure to ease gradually into the fast. Fasting as a tool should make your life better and bring about quality improvements, not give unnecessary restrictions to make your life difficult.

We also have to reiterate that you need to be sure you are in a state of perfect health before going about water fasting. Also, make sure you are under supervision if you intend to go for more extended periods of fasting. With this, we explore the various tips that could help you have smooth water fast.

Brace For the Fast

There is a saying that nothing good comes easy. Your decision to have a water fast is a decision to subject yourself to an exciting journey with some ups and downs. It is an adventure that will open you up to a fantastic experience that will reveal a lot about yourself and your body. Have it in mind that you are not facing the hangman, the executioner, the firing squad, or a death sentence.

This does not cancel out the fact that you are signing up for a challenge. However, consider this as a sacrifice you have to make to improve your overall health and well-being. The benefits of water fasting and autophagy are mouthwatering, which is more important than any temporary discomfort you might face.

Desist From Any Strenuous Activity

In other words, schedule the water fast during your free period. Bear in mind that you are not having any food during the time of the fast, so it is not a time to go about your regular activities. If it were an intermittent fast, you would be quite a bit more comfortable to go about your day as if nothing were happening.

However, with water fasting, you need to reserve your strength. Forget all personal or family demands. With this fast, you get to enjoy the period of rest without constant rumblings from your stomach.

Read

Be it a non-fiction book, a novel, or a magazine, books are the best friends to a faster. While you rest your body, it is vital to keep your mind occupied. With books, you can distract yourself from the hunger pangs and focus on what you are reading.

Besides, reading is not demanding. It is a low energy activity that can keep you engaged while you observe your fast.

Consider Short Fasting Periods

In other words, start small. In fact, you should not do any more than 24 hours of a water fast to start. If you decide to make water fasting a lifestyle, once a week is recommended. With this, you get to fast safely and be spared the stress that comes with long hours of fasting.

This does not mean you will not achieve your overall aim, be it autophagy or other benefits of water fasting.

Ease into the Fast

You have started reading about autophagy and its tremendous health benefits. The next day, you commence water fasting in a bid to allow your body to heal itself. No! It does not work that way. You are inviting disaster with this. Water fasting, an extreme form of fasting, is not the type for you nosedive into at all.

Instead, you have to prepare soundly. Have a transition period so that the sudden stoppage in the supply of food to your body does not cause extreme shock or adverse reactions. As a result, you have to gradually reduce your meals until you can comfortably thrive on the water for the number of days you decide to go with.

How everyone will ease into water fasting differs. Depending on the individual, it could be a couple of weeks to a month, depending on the advice from your health expert. The goal is to get the body prepared to survive on water and water only for the given number of days. This preparation, without a doubt, will not happen overnight.

In a bid to prepare your body for water fasting and ease into it, we prepare the next four-week plan:

Week 1: Avoid breakfast for the whole seven days. Make sure you are dedicated to this

Week 2: Eat only dinner and be sure to keep up with your water intake as well

Week 3: Still thriving on dinner only, reduce the ration you eat at night

Week 4: Try to start the water fast proper at this point.

In all the above, be sure to consume an adequate amount of water even while you skip meals. This can help keep the hunger pangs down.

Avoid Giving in to Hunger

Some of the advice above: reading a book, planning your fast, short fasting periods, etc., are all in a bid to reduce the effects of hunger. However, brace for hunger anyway while water fasting unless you are a veteran faster who is used to going for long periods without food. This is about the only way you might not feel so hungry.

However, there will be times when your stomach will become unruly. Drink a glass of water or two and have a nap to rest the hunger waves. This will reduce the hunger pangs, which will eventually disappear. Also, be sure NEVER to remain idle during the period of your fast. You need to keep your mind active to keep it off hunger.

Go Easy on Exercise

There are many reasons people choose to go for water fasting. However, we assume it is to activate the autophagy process in your body. Water fasting makes this process easy since there is no intake of calories in any form. You do not need to stress yourself with exercises.

If you must have a workout, be sure to limit it to less strenuous ones. Yoga is good, as it is not rigorous. Take a walk if you are not comfortable with yoga. The key is whatever will not make you expend too much energy.

Get Enough Rest

The importance of enough rest while water fasting cannot be overemphasized. Your body, your mind, and your emotions all need a break. You need this break, as water fasting drains you significantly, hence you have to conserve energy.

In addition to this is your sleep. Be sure to sleep well and follow a healthy sleep pattern. Avoid anything mentally tasking. Stay away from heavy machinery and driving. Your body will surely be giving you subtle signals. Pay close attention to this and follow all your body asks for well, except the cry to opt out. When you get a clue to sleep or take a nap, you need to do just that.

Take Time to Meditate

Meditation brings about a good and secure connection between your mind and body. Besides, it could prove as a very effective way to keep hunger pangs down, as well as reinforce your will-power.

Be Careful About Dizziness

There might be few instances of dizziness during water fasting. This might come up when you have been in a single position for too long and suddenly try to move. To take care of this, be sure not to rush things. Be it changing posture, rising from a seat or your bed, etc., taking in deep breaths before standing can be of great help. Should you feel dizzy, lie down or sit back down until the dizziness wears off.

Make sure you halt the fasting immediately if the dizziness persists, or you start to lose consciousness. This is part of why we recommend being under the supervision of a health practitioner while fasting.

Gradually Ease Out of the Fast

You have to be careful when breaking your water fast. We understand you are famished. You stood against all the odds and fought the cravings. This is not a license to gulp down whatever you feel like eating and rush every plate of food you get.

Instead, start with a juice to gradually bring your digestive system out of hibernation. Some minutes or hours later, introduce real food. Bear in mind that going without food has switched your body to the fasted state. Hence, it needs to gradually transition to the fed state via a small quantity of food. Make sure you only eat foods that can be digested easily, as well.

Stay Away from Junk

The idea behind water fasting in this book is to trigger autophagy, even though there might be other benefits like weight loss and many others. The idea here is that returning to your former, unhealthy eating habits will lead to a wasted effort.

While water fasting will give you a whole lot of health benefits, you have to support the effort with healthy food intake. Refined sugar, junk, and processed foods are all off the table.

Have Some Good Salts Available

As you go along the fast, you will need some electrolytes. You can get these via suitable quality salts like Himalayan Sea Salt or Redmond's

Real Salt. In the body, there is a hormone called insulin that will make sure the body cells get sugar and have the needed amount of sodium.

With reduced insulin levels, there will be an excess discharge of sodium from the body. This is expected in the first few days as the body adapts to the fast. Salts can also help you when you feel dizzy. A pinch of salt is all you need with some water. It can reset your body and cause an immediate change in mental function.

Avoid the Kitchen if Possible

Food cravings will hit you hard every time you go to the kitchen. Do yourself a favor and stay away from there. If possible, lock up the kitchen and get the key out of sight. This will help you stay on course while fasting. With time, your resilience grows, and you can dedicate yourself easily to the fast.

If you have to cook for your spouse or kids, be sure to have a nutritious cup of herbal tea available. You can sip this while preparing food. This will help reduce the cravings and nip the desire to eat.

Be Smart When Drinking Water

The periods in which the hunger sensation will come rushing at you are your regular feeding periods. This is expected, as it is a natural hormonal process where ghrelin, your hunger hormone, rises in a bid to drive you to eat. You can curb this by drinking water.

Herbal teas like chamomile and green tea are a good idea as well. Herbal tea has no calories, so you are not breaking any rule nor working against your effort to induce autophagy.

Consider a Sweet Drink

If you felt extremely down and drained as a result of the fast, you can attempt a calorie-free lemonade. You make this by adding organic lemon juice with liquid stevia mixed with water. With this, you get an improved mood that increases the feel-good neurotransmitters. This helps make the fast easy and enjoyable.

Doing this will surely bring about a noticeable improvement in your mood during the period of the fast. Besides, you get renewed vigor to handle the discomfort that comes with staying away from food. You do not need too much, because these drinks are really sweet and have no sugar or calories.

Many people have tried this and found it brought a soothing and calming effect, making them comfortable while they fasted. On the other hand, some people do not respond well to stevia. It does increase hunger and cravings in some people. This is a sign that it triggered insulin, and it is best to stay away from this if it happens.

Have a Spa Day

You are not eating for a couple of days. You have saved some money. You could invest in yourself in many ways. We recommend getting a massage or going to the spa and sauna. This is a proven way to reduce stress and get rid of excess toxins in your body. This will, at least, ease the fasting process.

Humans, by default, will move towards things that give pleasure. Food, without a doubt, does give pleasure. This explains why many people struggle with food addiction. This also explains why people are laden with a wide array of emotions during the early days of water fasting.

This is because the body has been configured to the neurochemical boost that comes from eating. Hence, it becomes a problem when the boost is absent.

Instead of the neurochemical boost from food, a spa day can be another positive reward your body looks forward to. Without a doubt, this will help suppress the variety of emotions that come forth as you fast. Going to the sauna is an exercise you will surely look forward to as you proceed with the water fast.

Get Grounded Daily

As much as possible, make it a duty to get outside daily and have your bare feet make contact with the ground, grass, or dirt. This is helpful, as there are some useful negative ions and healthy electromagnetic frequencies which serves as antioxidants that originate from the earth. We miss contact with these natural antioxidants because our shoe soles insulate us from the ground.

We recommend moving about barefoot in contact with the earth. This way, you get to ground the electromagnetic current originating from your body. This translates to mental clarity, relaxation, and improved energy. This is likened to taking a shower and getting rid of the EMFs you have on your body. Just like the good feeling we get after a bath, it is ideal, in the same way, to get rid of EMFs from your body by scheduling a specific period to get in contact with the earth.

While this is not compulsory for a successful fast, it will make your fast more enjoyable.

Get Daily Sunshine

Exposing large volume of your bare skin to the sun is pretty beneficial. This is not about burning your skin. Instead, you get some effective dose of vitamin D via a light suntan. This improves fat burning and helps you get into ketosis faster, paving the way for autophagy.

In addition to vitamin D, there are strong biophotons in the sunshine which serve as stress reducers. Alongside this, they help in the stimulation of feel good hormones: endorphins and dopamine, which will make fasting easier.

If you could subject yourself to the early morning sunshine, that would be great. Similar to getting grounded, it is not compulsory, but will surely help you have a smooth water fasting experience.

Final thoughts

Water fasting is one of the oldest and most powerful self-healing tools available to humanity. Without a doubt, it holds the key to a quick and tremendous health transformation guaranteed to reward you with abundant health benefits, including autophagy.

We, however, are not disputing the fact that water fasting could be pretty challenging, especially for first-timers. This is why we recommend taking essential steps to prepare yourself for a seamless fast. We have made these fantastic tips to reduce the toll the water fast will have on you.

With time, as you make fasting a lifestyle, you will get to a level where it becomes part of you such that the benefits come with ease, and without much stress.

Chapter 10:

How Long Until Autophagy Sets In

Many factors determine how long it will take for autophagy to set it. These range from the state of health of the person, to body fat percentage, to activity levels and more. Also, it depends on how much effort you are willing to invest in getting your body to autophagy.

There are many things to know about autophagy even though according to research, most of the signals occurs between mTOR and AMPK.

Mammalian Target of Rapamycin, or mTOR, is the primary nutrient regulator in the body, which you might recall from an earlier chapter. It is responsible for cellular growth, anabolism, and protein synthesis. It encourages the activation of insulin receptors and the formation of new tissue.

AMP-activated protein kinase, or AMPK, is a fuel sensor that helps bring a balance to the body when the energy level is low by fostering homeostasis and triggering the backup fuel of the body.

MTOR works against autophagy, as it encourages growth in the body while AMPK promotes autophagy as a result of the consumption of internal energy stores and lower energy state. When the body does not have enough nutrients, AMPK works against the growth of cells by reducing mTORC1 pathway. This gives the body no option but to break down the weakest components.

What Stops Autophagy?

The lower the levels of a number of body nutrients such as glucose, calories, and amino acids, the more the need for autophagy. Ideally, the body is not really motivated to turn on stored energy and body tissue to recycle it. However, under the right conditions, this happens.

When there are enough food nutrients in the body, both AMPK and mTOR sense it. This calls for a decision among the body cells whether to foster growth or switch to autophagy. Other growth factors such as IGF-1, insulin, and mechanical muscle stimuli also determine which takes place.

By default, some things will work against switching the body to autophagy and all its associated process. These are:

IGF-1 and insulin point to the presence of anabolic nutrients that foster growth. This triggers the Akt/mTORC1/p70S6K pathway in the body, causing the synthesis of muscle protein. This is precisely what autophagy is trying to achieve.

Carbs, which raise blood sugar and insulin, will stop autophagy. Even though your body is breaking down nutrients alongside inactive mTOR while consuming carbs, autophagy will be impossible since those two nutrients are present.

The body will not see the reason to activate autophagy with amino acids and proteins. This is because the body interprets this as an abundance of essential nutrients. There can be reduced protein intake such that there will not be a breakdown of muscle protein. However, as long as you feed on protein, autophagy will likely not take place due to the presence of a protein that triggers mTOR. This explains why restricting protein does not adequately help activate autophagy.

Too many calories from macronutrients will work against autophagy. When there are excess amounts of carbs, exogenous ketones, fats, or protein in the body, it raises mTOR and insulin, which in turn reduces AMPK. While insulin levels will not spike so much when consuming fat, it will be stored. The body, as a result of this, considers autophagy unnecessary.

All in all, it is good to consider autophagy as dependent on the status of the nutrients of your body cells. This means the number of amino acids they get access to, the level of your blood sugar, how nourished your blood sugar level is, the last time you fed as well as the rate at which you expend energy at the moment.

Fasting for Autophagy: How Long?

While discussing the chapter on water fasting, we recommend a maximum of 72 hours to fast. This is because all you need to activate autophagy via fast is a 48 to 72 hour fast. This is how long it takes to get to ketosis, when the body commences the production of ketone bodies.

It is important to point out at this juncture that there is no reliable way of measuring the rate of autophagy in humans. However, it can be estimated by considering the glucose ketone index as well as the insulin to glucose ratio.

When the insulin to glucose ratio is low, it is pointing to a lot of breakdown of nutrients, fat oxidations, gluconeogenesis, and ketogenesis.

When the insulin to glucagon ratio is high, it suggests increased blood sugar, nutrient storage, and more anabolism.

When the glucose ketone index gives an insulin-glucagon ratio that has a low score, this points to increased AMPK and higher ketosis.

The duration it takes for autophagy to set in is a factor of your body nutrients, as well as the presence of some nutrients in your body like glucose, ketones, and amino acids. If you have conditioned your body not to consume excess fats and protein daily, getting into autophagy will be more comfortable and faster, compared to someone that will have to burn a lot of these calories initially.

How Long Before Autophagy Sets In

With excess carbs and protein, it will take a longer fasting duration for the body to trigger autophagy. This is why a protein fast is one of the ways to get to autophagy. Not only this, consuming too many calories, way more than the body needs, will increase how long it will take the body to trigger autophagy.

This explains why you need to restrict the amount of calories you take in. This is especially important if you care about longevity, as it conditions the body such that getting into autophagy comes fast and easy. As a result, your fasting period will not be too long before you reap the associated benefits.

A couple of things that make autophagy come faster are:

Fasting and concentrating on zero calorie meals is the best and most effective way to activate autophagy. Water fasting, intermittent fasting, and other forms of fasting reduce blood sugar levels, insulin, mTOR, and sieves out glucose and amino acids in the liver.

You can also restrict calories without fasting. You get to experience autophagy faster when you fast overnight as well. Since the intake of amino acids into your system is paused, getting into autophagy will be fast during the period when you are without food.

You can also restrict protein to stimulate autophagy, which works better than restricting carbs or fats. The con with this, however, is the tendency of the person to experience muscle loss. With intermittent fasting, you can get the benefits of restricting calories on autophagy. A prolonged fast duration accompanied by an intake of enough nutrients like protein will promote intense autophagy, which will guard against unwanted muscle loss.

With exercise and resistance training, you get to increase the level of AMPK, which helps autophagy. When you work out, the body uses amino acids and glycogen, which makes it more comfortable to get into autophagy. In the body, there are mechanical stimuli that also activate mTOR which inhibits autophagy. However, it is inside the muscle cell, and not the liver, that the significant activation of mTOR takes place. This sustains macroautophagy in the liver, brain, kidney, and other body tissues, which is where it is supposed to be.

The primary assignment of mTOR should be to build nerve and muscle cells, and not tumors or fat cells. The right place for autophagy as well is the brain and liver, not the muscle. Resistance training coupled with fasting is the best combination to derive benefits from autophagy and mTOR while dodging the side effects of an excess of both.

Determining when autophagy will set in is not black and white because you first have to ascertain the number of days it will take you to get to ketosis.

The speed of getting into autophagy is a factor of many things like the metabolic state of the person, nutrient status, energy requirements, and overall health. A person who eats a regulated amount of carbs and has very low blood glucose and insulin can activate autophagy faster. On the other hand, a person taking in hundreds of grams per day will take pretty long, the same way it will take someone on a high protein diet.

Whatever the state of the body, one thing is sure; there will be some period of fasting before you can drain the body of glucose and amino acids.

- Consider a standard Western diet that typically contains an approximation of 50% carb, 15% protein, and 35% fat. People in this category will need no less than 72 hours of fasting to activate ketosis and autophagy.

- A low carb, moderate protein diet will need 24 hours of fasting to get to autophagy.

- On a low carb, high protein diet as well, you will need more than 24 hours of fasting for autophagy. However, you will likely experience autophagy between meals.

- For a low carb, low protein diet with few calories, there is a high probability of autophagy between 20 hours of fasting. It is also possible between meals even though for active autophagy, you will have to fast for a longer period and eat adequate nutrients.

- A high carb, low protein diet should get you to autophagy within 24 hours of fasting. There is however, a high chance of muscle breakdown.

- A high carb moderate protein diet will need about 2 to 3 days of fasting before autophagy sets in. This is because of the abundant nutrients that have to be burned.

The idea is equipping the body with the needed nutrients such as fatty acids, amino acids, vitamins, and minerals without excess dependence on calories that are not required. Excess calories will make it pretty difficult for the body to keep the metabolism running as it should.

Whatever the diet you plan to go with, bear in mind that fasting, intermittent fasting and water fasting, is the best path to foster your way to autophagy.

Chapter 11:

Autophagy: Can It Ever Be In Excess?

In case you are worried about a lack or excess of autophagy, this chapter will answer your questions by shedding light on the optimal amount of autophagy that is recommended for humans.

Why is Autophagy Crucial?

Of all the ways of promoting lifespan in man and animal, restricting calories is the most acceptable. This, however, does not mean you have to starve to live long.

Not at all.

Many benefits come from autophagy, which is also promoted through calorie restriction. Animals that do not experience autophagy do not live long, even if they reduce the number of calories they consume. In other words, autophagy must be sufficient to reap the benefits of calorie restriction.

Without adequate autophagy, aging and other associated disease are inevitable. This is why autophagy is the key to controlling muscle loss, promoting insulin sensitivity, reducing inflammation, getting rid of waste materials, and getting into ketosis.

Unwanted Side Effects of Autophagy to Keep in Mind

- Sadly, some tumors and cancer cells can thrive even with autophagy
- Excessive autophagy will trigger muscle loss

- There are some bacterial infection that comes around due to autophagy

- Ideally, have in mind that when malignant tumor cells are subjected to nutritional stress via reduced calorie intake or fasting, such cells might not die because autophagy inhibits apoptosis.

- While autophagy is very good in the control of disease, it might not be the best bet for treatment. This is why autophagy should be controlled.

- Many people do not naturally experience autophagy, and the kind of lifestyle they lead makes it impossible for them ever to experience it. This calls for controlled water fasting along with exercise.

Autophagy: Is There an Optimum Amount?

There is no precise figure that expresses the optimum level of autophagy a person can experience. This is due to the abundant variables, and the fact that humans differ in many ways. Many things affect the level of autophagy processes. Some of these are the level of physical activity, your present medical condition, the amount of food you eat, your current state of metabolism, and overall health situation.

There is no fixed value for the amount of optimal autophagy, and it keeps changing. Some things will tell you if you need more or less autophagy. Some of these are your biomarkers, your current well-being, your relationship with food, and your sleep quality.

The table below explains situations or conditions where you might benefit from more or less autophagy, depending on various factors we examined above. The next section will explore in detail conditions that make you want to have more or less autophagy.

More Autophagy	More fasting	Less fasting, more calories	Less Autophagy
If you are overweight	High Blood Pressure	If you have low thyroid	Cancer
If you are pre-diabetic	High Insulin and IGF-1	If you have muscle loss and sarcopenia	Bacterial Infection
High Triglycerides	Addicted to eating or other eating disorders	If you are underweight	
High Inflammation		If you are underage	

When Do You Need More Autophagy

There are times you need more fasting to activate more autophagy.

Insulin Resistance

If you have pre-diabetes or other signs of insulin resistance, frequent fasting can help trigger autophagy, which causes healing. This is because people with excess fats are subjected to defective hepatic autophagy, which fosters endoplasmic reticulum stress alongside insulin resistance. A 72 hour fast can cause a 50% drop in insulin levels for people in this category.

You Suffer from Obesity

Excess calories in the body are stored as body fat. This is a good source of energy that the body can turn to when fasting. This is why fasting is the easiest way for people who are overweight to shed off unwanted pounds and slim down.

You are Prone to Alzheimer's

Autophagy is central to maintaining balance in the brain and intracellular homeostasis. When mice lose autophagy, they begin to have protein aggregates and neurodegeneration. Autophagy can be likened to a waste disposal system that gets rid of these aggregates from the nervous system. People who show signs of Alzheimer's experience deficiency in autophagy.

Traumatic Brain Injury

You need to protect your neurons against death after a brain injury. This, alongside the maintenance of cellular homeostasis, is possible with autophagy. A ketogenic diet alongside exogenous ketones will also energize the brain.

Presence of Skin Rashes or Breakouts

Autophagy helps against inflammation and oxidative stress response. It controls and regulates the production of inflammatory pathologies in the body.

Other cases in which you need more autophagy are excessive body fat, high blood sugar levels, excessive inflammation, metabolic syndrome, and an unhealthy relationship with food.

When Do You Need Less Autophagy?

There are other conditions when you need less autophagy. Some of these are:

You Lead an Active Lifestyle

One of the ways to boost autophagy is exercise. Hence, if you are already active physically, you already reap the benefits of autophagy. If you combine exercise with reduced calories, there is a high probability you will lose muscle and also have reduced performance.

If you fast, you might notice reduced energy along with weakness. This is a clue to take a step back, as you need more nutrients to compensate for your active lifestyle.

You are Underweight

If you are already skinny or you have lost muscle, it is better you concentrate on feeding yourself and getting the required nutrients. Be sure to get enough calories and reduce your fasting window.

You Have a Physical Injury

For you to heal and your body to repair damaged body tissue, essential food nutrients are very important. Even though autophagy and fasting will promote quick recovery and take care of the inflammation, you need enough sleep, calories, healthy fats, and collagen for adequate healing.

You Have a Malignant Disease

There are malignant diseases with which constant fasting is not the best approach to take care of them. Without a doubt, autophagy does help to suppress tumors in the initial stage of tumorigenesis. With time, however, it could enhance the propagation of the tumor. Malignancy should be treated with oxygen therapy and a keto diet.

You Suffer from Hypothyroidism

Fasting slows down the metabolic rate, being a stressor that reduces thyroid hormones. Hence, if you suffer from this, you need less fasting and more of the foods that boost thyroids.

You are Pregnant or Breastfeeding

If you are pregnant, you do not need extended periods of fasting. Besides, your meals should be full of high-quality nutrients. You can practice intermittent fasting without extended fasting periods.

You are Elderly

According to research, autophagy can help maintain muscle mass and guard against age-related muscle dysfunction. As you grow older, however, there is a big chance that your body starts resisting anabolic hormone and nutrients. This calls for increased protein as well as reduced fasting windows, because seniors are more susceptible to frailty and sarcopenia.

You are Underage

Young folks under the age of 15 need not subject themselves to any extended fasting window. This is perfectly healthy as long as they do not have an unhealthy relationship with food. Spiking insulin levels occurring many times a day make one the right candidate for pre-diabetes. As a result of this, it is essential to teach your kids healthy eating habits. Folks above 16 years could experiment with intermittent fasting.

If you experience hair loss, bone fractures, constantly feeling cold, issues falling asleep, low energy levels, and less body fat, you need less autophagy.

Final Thoughts

As fabulous as the benefits of autophagy are, taking steps to induce it is not for everyone. We have seen from the above that there are some categories of people that will not benefit too much from autophagy. Be sure to know the category you fall into and work along with it appropriately.

Chapter 12:
Lifestyle and Foods That Help
With Autophagy

When people hear about autophagy, all that comes to their mind is fasting and exercise to activate it. These are, however, not the only ways to activate autophagy.

It is not until you stay away from food for 3 to 5 days that you get to see the benefits of autophagy. Getting into autophagy is a factor of what you do before, during, and after the fast. Besides this, there are many other ways you can activate and speed autophagy up.

We have explained in detail how to boost autophagy using exercise, intermittent fasting, water fasting, and the ketogenic diet in earlier chapters. To avoid repetition, we will skip those and explore other means through which you can activate and speed up autophagy. Our recommendations, after a series of research, are based on lifestyle changes and healthy foods that can make the autophagy process come fast enough. Even your sleep habits, as you will see from the first point, can help activate autophagy.

Circadian Rhythm, Melatonin, and Deep Sleep

Getting adequate, deep, and high-quality sleep is not negotiable if you want to activate autophagy. Poor sleep habits and patterns do hurt cognitive function. Besides, if you do not sleep well at night, or if your sleep is characterized by constant waking up incessantly through the night, the process of autophagy will be affected.

As a result, the length and quality of your sleep is significant. This is why you should strive for seven hours of deep sleep every night. There are many things you can do to improve your sleep, such as:

- Take a warm shower before bed
- Drink a glass of milk before bed
- Ensure a well ventilated and relaxed atmosphere
- Reduce or get rid of all sources of light, especially blue light and screens, from your room. The presence of light decreases neurogenesis, which also affects cognitive performance. If you use an alarm, be sure the light from the screen is any other color besides blue
- Have a fixed sleep schedule and stick to it
- Your last meal should come at least three hours before going to bed. If you have to eat, only have foods that are easy to digest like the ones recommended above and MCT oil, bone broth, and raw honey.
- Set your circadian rhythm by exposing your eyes to the early morning sun
- Do not watch films that will get you excited or worked up before bed. If possible, avoid TV during the last hour of your day.
- Stay away from caffeine in the afternoon. Depending on the person, some people will have to avoid caffeine after 2 pm while others will be later in the afternoon. Caffeine makes the quality of sleep suffer.
- Stay away from all forms of stress before going to bed. If possible, practice deep breathing, a five-minute meditation, or whatever relaxation technique works for you.

- Alcohol is a no-no before bed, as it will prevent you from experiencing deep sleep. You want deep sleep, as that is what heals the brain and body.

- Melatonin secretion is also affected by the presence of EMF. Turn off Wi-Fi, mobile devices, and other electronic gadgets you have in your bedroom.

- Completely black out your room. You can use a sleep mask overnight to help with this.

The idea is to do all you can to ensure you trigger the secretion and release of melatonin at night. This will help maintain your circadian rhythm and help you get better sleep quality.

According to research, our circadian rhythm, which is the sleep-wake cycle, also controls autophagy and affects cognitive function (Kondratova, 2012).

The pineal gland, a small gland located in the brain, releases melatonin, a type of hormone. This hormone is in charge of the circadian rhythm. The body needs optimum levels of melatonin to fall asleep and ensure deep sleep through the night.

According to research, melatonin induces autophagy in the brain and helps guard against neuropsychiatric disorders. Our circadian rhythm is so delicate that slight changes in the environment can disturb it and work against melatonin production which reduces autophagy and affects our cognition.

Cold and Hot Exposure

Getting exposed to both hot and cold temperature can also help trigger autophagy. This is because it stresses the cells. There is research that revealed the fact that you can trigger autophagy via heat stress (Dokladny, 2015). Besides this, there is a relationship between the heat shock response and autophagy.

According to research, you also start neuronal autophagy via exposure to cold, which can lower the risk of neurodegenerative diseases (Aihara, 2016).

- Switching back and forth between cold and hot temperatures can also trigger autophagy. How can you apply this in your daily life?
- Try to alternate between a hot and cold shower
- Spend time in a sauna and immediately go for a cold shower
- You can also take a walk during winter with little clothes and directly come home and have a hot shower.
- You can also expose yourself to cold via cold plunges and cold baths.

Hyperbaric Oxygen Therapy

Also known as HBOT, Hyperbaric oxygen therapy is a treatment used to foster healing and recovery of the body cells and central nervous system after an injury. This is why some patients are subjected to oxygen chambers after an injury.

In the body, oxygen is transported strictly through the red blood cells. With HBOT, however, oxygen gets dissolved in all body fluids, the ones of the central nervous system included. As a result of this, most, if not all, parts of the body where blood circulation is blocked get oxygen. This ensures that damaged tissues, as well as body parts that have to heal, have oxygen.

Some studies claim that HBOT helps elevate and enhance autophagy in the central nervous system (Liu, 2017). This is best done with the help of an expert, though. It should be pointed out that HBOT can be expensive. But a viable alternative is via the use of oxygen concentrators, which is cheaper and pretty readily available compared to HBOT.

Acupuncture

This is an alternative treatment that is proven to induce autophagy in the brain (Tian, 2016). According to a study, acupuncture improves memory and learning, which also protects brain cells, which happens by upregulating the autophagy pathway (HD, 2016).

Acupuncture is useful and helpful if you are willing to try it out. Auricular acupuncture in particular involves inserting needles in the ears. You can find health practitioners who provide this.

There are also acupuncture mats that can also help you relax before going to bed.

Foods that Induce Autophagy

In addition to fasting and other lifestyle changes, some healthy food choices can help trigger autophagy. A few of these are discussed below.

Coffee and Caffeine

Coffee is also one of the most significant ways to trigger autophagy in the brain. According to research, both regular and decaffeinated coffee help trigger autophagy (Pietrocola, 2014). Coffee contains a compound known as polyphenols, which also protects the brain because it fosters autophagy.

Studies on caffeine have revealed that caffeine also keeps the brain cells in good condition and reduces the risk of developing neurodegenerative conditions by triggering autophagy (Luan, 2018). A cup of coffee every morning is a good idea.

However, as explained above, stay away from coffee later in the day, as it disrupts sleep. Ideally, your last cup of coffee should be around noon if you want a good night's sleep.

It is also recommended that you consume the entire coffee fruit rather than pure caffeine or coffee beans. Research has established that having a whole coffee fruit concentrate increases brain function.

Green Tea

Epigallocatechin-3-Gallate (EGCG), the major polyphenol found in green tea, has been shown to have neuroprotective and anti-inflammatory effects.

EGCG is a good compound that triggers brain autophagy and guards the brain cells against toxicity. It does also helps take care of neurodegenerative conditions.

Green tea can also help to improve memory and learning, as it restores autophagic flux in the brain, especially after chronic stress.

Coconut Oil and Medium Chain Triglycerides (MCTs)

One of the best brain foods you can take is coconut oil. Not only does it work to support your thyroid, it increases ketone levels, thereby stimulating autophagy.

One or two tablespoons of coconut oil per day is a good idea. Coconut oil has medium-chain triglycerides (MCTs) which boost the ketone production effect of coconut oil.

Broccoli Sprouts (Sulforaphane)

Cruciferous vegetables like Brussels sprouts, broccoli, cabbage, kale, and cauliflower contain sulforaphane, which is a phytochemical. This sulforaphane has antioxidant and anti-inflammatory properties just like curcumin.

Research has shown that sulforaphane boosts autophagy in the brain cells (Sun, 2018). This is why it is very useful in combating neurodegenerative diseases. Sulforaphane can be taken both in the form of a supplement or via broccoli sprouts.

Galangal

This is a spice which is also known as "Siamese ginger" or "Thai ginger" because it takes the form of ginger. It is an exotic spice that is common in Malaysia, Indonesia, and Thailand.

Inside galangal is a compound known as galangin, which triggers autophagy and keeps the brain neuron cells protected.

Extra Virgin Olive Oil (Oleuropein)

There are many health benefits of olive oil, and it is well known for its anti-inflammatory effects. Inside olive oil is a polyphenol known as oleuropein which induces autophagy and also takes care of cognitive impairment.

A diet rich in extra virgin oil will induce autophagy, making it very effective for the treatment of Alzheimer's in patients. You can also take olive oil without adding it to anything.

Reishi Mushroom

Reishi mushroom is a pretty potent fungus with many bioactive compounds. For thousands of years, it has been used by Chinese medicine practitioners to serve as a boost for the immune system, to regulate inflammation, reduce inflammation, and boost brain health.

Research has also established that reishi mushrooms can activate autophagy (Rosario-Acevedo, 2013). It also regulates autophagy, thus keeping the brain cells in good condition.

Turmeric (Curcumin)

This is the spice responsible for the yellow color of curry. It is a natural compound that protects the brain cells from damage by paving the way for the autophagy process.

Berries

Berries in various forms such as strawberries, blueberries, and acai berries are all recommended. They contain phenol which helps activate autophagy and keeps the brain cells protected from oxidative stress and inflammation. Berries also help to improve cognitive function.

Omega-3 Fatty Acids

The body cannot produce and store Omega-3 fatty acids, yet they are essential fatty acids which are important for normal functioning of the brain and central nervous system.

Omega-3 fatty acids, according to research, help reduce brain inflammation, improve mood, memory, and cognition (Pearson, 2017). It also protects against dementia, Alzheimer's disease, and other forms of mild cognitive impairment.

Research has also shown that omega-3 fatty acids foster BDNF signaling which helps with brain autophagy. You can get Omega-3 fatty acids from seafood and cold water fish like:

- Black cod
- Sardines
- Sablefish
- Salmon
- Herring

Aside from helping with autophagy, these are essential brain foods that will keep your cognitive function in top condition. Many people are deficient in omega-3 fatty acids. It can, however, be gotten in the form of supplement by using krill oil – a distinct type of fish oil with the essential omega-3 fatty acids.

Supplements to Induce Autophagy

In addition to the above food choices, there are other natural supplements that do induce autophagy. We discuss a couple of them below:

American GInseng

American Ginseng is a pretty potent supplement that promotes brain autophagy. It reduces mitochondrial dysfunction and protects the brain from neurotoxicity through autophagy.

It also helps treat neurodegenerative disorders and helps with improving mental clarity. Users can get this in optimal ketones supplements.

Ginkgo Biloba

This is a Chinese herb that has been used for thousands of years to address a number of health issues. It is one of the most natural supplements prescribed as an herb around the world.

It is known to improve blood flow, mood, mental clarity, memory, and give an overall improvement of the brain health in many individuals. It greatly lowers the risk of dementia and Alzheimer's disease. Its ability to activate brain autophagy makes it a very good treatment for these diseases, as well.

Acetyl-L-Carnitine

Also known as ALCAR, this is an amino acid and carnitine that has been acetylated. According to research, it protects the neurons and enhances cognitive functions (Toxnet, 2018). It also increases mental sharpness and alertness, thereby boosting brain health. It also helps get rid of serious fatigue and improves your mood.

It also induces autophagy in the brain, thereby encouraging mitochondria function and guarding against cognitive decline. In simple terms, it makes you strong and resilient.

Vitamin D

This is a fat soluble vitamin synthesized by the skin on exposure to the sun. Many people are, however, deficient in this vitamin.

This could be an issue because almost every body tissue has vitamin D receptors. Thus, a deficiency could trigger some consequences, both psychological and physiological. According to research, the activation of vitamin D and vitamin D receptors triggers autophagy (Wu, 2011).

There is research that points out that deficiency of vitamin D leads to diseases that involve a lack of autophagy (Somma, 2017). All you need to get vitamin D is to expose yourself to the early morning sun. However, many people do not get this, especially during the winter. There are vitamin D sunlamps and vitamin D supplements as well that you can use.

Lithium

Generally, lithium is a medication used by bipolar patients to manage their condition. It is an essential mineral which, when introduced in small doses, could improve brain health, trigger the formation of myelin, and induce autophagy.

It also triggers the breakdown of the protein which is responsible for neurodegenerative and neuropsychiatric diseases. As a result, it is a good treatment for dementia, Parkinson's disease, Alzheimer's disease, and Huntington's disease.

Cannabidiol (CBD)

Found in marijuana, it is an active cannabinoid. It is, however, not psychoactive and will not make you high. It is a good treatment for a number of conditions because of its effect on inflammation.

According to research, CBD oil induces autophagy pathways in the brain (Maroon, 2018). It can help reduce stress and help you sleep well.

Rhodiola

Also known as Arctic root or golden root, Rhodiola is a traditional Scandinavian and Chinese herb. It is a popular adaptogen that can help improve mental and physical stamina. It also induces autophagy and helps reduce degeneration of brain neurons.

Based on research, Rhodiola does help significantly upregulate autophagy.

Berberine

This is an alkaloid that comes from various plants. It comes with anti-inflammatory properties and helps protect the neurons and also guard against depression. It helps lower cholesterol and improve intestinal health.

Berberine boosts autophagy, reduces inflammation, and protects the brain from damage. According to a study, berberine promotes neurogenesis and reduces neurological deficits by enhancing autophagy (Zhang, 2016).

Nicotinamide

Also known as nicotinic acid amide or niacinamide, it is a water soluble form of vitamin B3, the very active type. It is a good component that helps combat the thriving of Alzheimer's disease and also enhances cognitive function.

By enhancing brain autophagy, it reduces cognitive decline, thereby preserving mitochondrial integrity.

Schisandra

This is a berry common among the Traditional Chinese Medical Practitioners. It has seeds containing lignin that come with many health promoting properties. Traditionally, it is used to treat stress, depression, and menopause.

Research indicates that people struggling with Alzheimer's disease and Parkinson's disease can also benefit from Schisandra. This is due to its ability to limit degeneration of neurons and cognitive impairment by fostering autophagy.

It also protects the brain neurons and guards against inflammation in the brain cell. It is available in powders and pills.

Spermidine

This is a polyamine compound that comes with a lot of metabolic functions. It can be gotten in living tissues and a wide range of foods like cheese, chicken, fermented soy, potatoes, and pears. It is also available in supplement form.

It has a protective effect on the neurons, enhances autophagy, and reduces synapses aging (Bhukel, 2017). Due to its anti degenerative effect on the neurons, it enhances cognitive functions, reduces memory impairment, and guards neurons from demyelination.

Chapter 13:

Common Autophagy Mistakes to Avoid

In trying to get to autophagy, there are some errors that might work against your efforts. A knowledge of these errors will keep you on the right path to make sure you are doing the right thing. Due to the effectiveness of autophagy in promoting health, longevity, and well-being, it has gained wide acceptance. It is not surprising that many people will have come up with different ideas about the concept. Thus, if you are not well grounded in the topic, it is easy to fall for some beliefs that could turn out to be errors which could hinder autophagy.

So far, we have explored many ways of activating autophagy. Of all the methods discussed, the most effective and reliable way is prolonged fasting (water fasting or intermittent fasting) and a practice of calorie restriction. The aim of this is to make nutrients scarce in the body such that the body has no choice but to recycle old cells.

While there is no known way to measure autophagy, it has been accepted that low insulin levels, deficiency of glucose, and amino acids all suppress mTOR which provides a fertile ground for autophagy. Excess levels of AMPK also support autophagy.

Autophagy Mistakes to Keep in Mind

When it comes to autophagy, there is still much to learn about the process. However, we can identify some mistakes to avoid when trying to induce autophagy:

- Anything that raises your insulin level and spikes your blood sugar will stop autophagy
- Excessive nutrients in the body does not support autophagy
- Fasting and staying away from food promotes autophagy
- Maintaining a lower insulin to glucagon ratio promotes autophagy
- Irregular eating supports autophagy

If your goal is to harness the self healing power of autophagy, enjoy the longevity boosting effect and all that it has to offer, watch out for the following mistakes in trying to get to autophagy.

Inadequate Fasting Duration

For you to activate autophagy, you need to be ready to fast for 3 to 5 days. However, the exact duration depends on the specific individual and the balance between the person's mTOR and AMPK. Many people hold onto the belief that with an intermittent fasting duration of between 12 and 16 hours, they can activate autophagy and get rid of cancer cells, boost their growth hormones, and release their stem cells.

The plain truth, however, is that a 16 hour fast is too small to get your body into a real fasted state. This is because:

- Fasting does not begin immediately when you stop eating your last meal. You will have to digest the nutrients first and until the nutrients are digested, you have not started fasting.
- After your last meal, you still need about four hours for the post absorptive state

As a result of the above, you need about five to six hours after eating before you can get to the fasted state. The body is still actively burning the calories from food you have ingested.

With the above in mind, to really get to autophagy, brace for a fast duration of more than 24 hours. Ideally, a 3 to 5 day fast is recommended.

Fatty Coffee

Bear in mind that fats will not raise your insulin levels the way proteins or carbs will. They will, however, raise your mTOR level and put you in the feasted state.

During the period of our forefathers, it was easy for ketone bodies to induce macroautophagy and chaperone-mediated autophagy as a result of excessive starvation. You can get this effect again by adding ketone boosting fats, like MCT oil, to your coffee.

The problem, however, is that excessive fat will enhance your insulin level and raise mTOR which will break your fast. This is why we recommend just a teaspoon of ketone boosting fats.

To be sure you are on a smooth path to autophagy, try and stay away from calories and its sources. We would not even recommend MCT oil in your coffee unless you want to extend your fast and need some to boost energy along the way.

Taking BCAAs

Also known as Branched-Chain Amino Acids, these are constituents of pure amino acids that stops autophagy with ease.

Many people, in a bid to guard against muscle loss do take BCAA. This fear is, however, not justified, because prolonged fasting and ketosis will prevent the breakdown of muscles because of the growth hormones and surplus ketone bodies.

If you take BCAA, however, it gets you off ketosis thereby stopping autophagy. This might eventually cause the breakdown of muscle and tissue cells. Also, taking BCAA has been associated with mood disorders and some neurotransmitter imbalances. As a result, it is a good idea to stay away from BCAA unless you truly need it.

If you are doing a fasted workout, you can take BCAA as the body is synthesizing protein and mTOR.

Taking Artificial Sweeteners

There are calories that claim to be zero calorie sweeteners. The issue with these sweeteners is that they can raise insulin in the cephalic phase response, which makes the gut release insulin.

Ordinarily, thinking of, seeing, or even smelling food raises your appetite level which fosters the release of insulin and gastric juices even before you eat. You have the food sensation which makes your intestines and digestive system prepare for these nutrients by releasing insulin in readiness.

Common artificial sweeteners like saccharin, aspartame, and sucralose raise blood and insulin levels in a group of people. Stevia and erythritol also could be culprits.

The key is knowing the effect of artificial sweeteners on your blood level and the response your body gives. All in all, bear in mind that artificial sweeteners will likely mess with autophagy and affect gut microbes, hence if your aim is activating autophagy, stay away from them for the time being.

You Supplement with Calories

Many supplements are available that come with sugar and extra calories that can easily break a fast. There are others as well with reasonable calorie amounts that are pretty safe.

Krill oil capsules or vitamin D are low in fat and if you do not take more than 2 servings, they will neither break your fast nor affect autophagy. There are other herbal supplements like berberine, turmeric, or mushroom complex which do not affect autophagy either.

The problem starts when you start taking too many supplements. Excessive supplements will add up to excessive calories that can break a fast. This is why supplements are a bad idea while fasting.

If your fast is between a week, you do not really need supplements as you will hardly become nutrient deficient. If you must take a supplement, however, consider magnesium and potassium chloride.

Discrepancy in Your Circadian Rhythm

Without deep sleep, it is rare to activate autophagy. Growth hormones occur in the same way and are released between the hours of 11 pm and 2 am.

As a result, if you desire to get the best of autophagy, we recommend going to bed earlier and getting a deep restful sleep as early as possible. This is when any major physical repair takes place.

Your calorie restriction or the length of your fast do not matter if you are not getting quality sleep. It is during sleep that you get real benefits of autophagy and the growth hormones.

Not Having Extended Fasting Periods

You cannot expect to have any real and impactful autophagy if your fasting period is not more than 24 hours. Even if you get to activate autophagy briefly, you might just be there for a couple of minutes which will not translate to any significant health benefit.

In this regard, we recommend time restricted eating as a daily habit to get the body to a state of low insulin and reduced mTOR. However, real autophagy comes when you stay away from food for extended periods.

At least once a month, aim to stay away from food for three to five days. Get clear with your schedule and make this a habit to get the real benefits of autophagy.

Frequent Long Fasting

Excessive fasting that activates too much autophagy is not a good idea either, because it comes with some side effects.

The signs of too much fasting are pretty easy to detect. When you start feeling weak and drained, lose muscle mass, etc., this points to excessive fasting. Even though you want the benefits of autophagy, you have to nourish your body.

If you are overweight, then it is normal to fast excessively without any associated side effects. With more body fat, extended fasting becomes easier without any pronounced side effects. People who are lean and physically active need not fast too much.

It is also important to prioritize frequency and consistency of fasting. Having a fasting schedule and eating junk the rest of the times does not make any sense.

In fact, it is better to have short periods of fasting once in a while than stress your body with long fasts and packing in junk along with other unhealthy habits.

Eating Too Little Food Nutrients

It is a bad idea to fast for long and not eat anything tangible when it is time to break that fast. While this might be helpful from a caloric point of view, overall health gets jeopardized.

Fasting in itself decreases the amount of food nutrients that get into the body. As a result of this, getting adequate food nutrients is pretty important.

Be sure to concentrate on nutrient dense foods like wild fish, beef, pastured eggs, organ meats, herbs, spices, vegetables, low carb berries, organ meats, and fruits.

Concentrating on fast foods or low carb meals will not give you the essential micronutrients. This calls for concentration on high quality food.

Not Getting Adequate Workouts

While fasting is a pretty powerful tool to activate autophagy, it is only part of the equation. You still have to be smart with your sleep, exercise, and nutrition.

If you are fasting, endeavor to add low impact exercise. In the same manner, supplement your workout with some form of intermittent fasting.

Exercise coupled with restricted training is another tested way of inducing autophagy and getting the associated health benefits.

Many people fast without exercising. The problem with this, however, is that you will not reach your maximum health potential. A combination of both brings optimum results.

Final Thoughts

All in all, autophagy is not a phenomenon for a restricted set of people. Once you keep the above mistakes in mind, you can easily prepare a fertile ground for autophagy to take place. Bear in mind that the foundation is restricted eating and adequate exercise, coupled with the right sleep pattern and staying away from some food items.

Knowledge of these mistakes will go a long way in guarding you against making any silly mistake that might work against your efforts.

Conclusion

So far so good! It is evident that autophagy holds the key to improved health, longevity, and overall sound living. This manual has discussed extensively all you have to know about autophagy. We have examined the ways in which you can activate autophagy. Even if you have a phobia of fasting, there are other life choices you can make to prepare your body for autophagy.

Without a doubt, autophagy holds tremendous health benefits for humans. However, as encouraging, exciting, and beneficial as the health benefits of autophagy are, it is not for everyone. We have analyzed the category of people who will not benefit from autophagy and looked at whether or not there is such a thing as excess autophagy or too little autophagy.

Autophagy is good. But when it occurs in excess, it could do more harm than good. When do you want more autophagy to take place, and when will autophagy result in other unwanted side effects? Be sure to get familiar with the pages of this book to determine which one suits you.

You could have unknowingly held on to some misconceptions about autophagy. These were so-called facts that you have been fed by the media or other so called autophagy experts. We dedicated a chapter to debunking many untrue beliefs that people have held onto over the years about autophagy. A knowledge of these will help you know what to truly expect from it.

Over the course of this book, we emphasized many times that the best way to get into autophagy is via staying away from food for long periods and exercising. There is a chapter dedicated to water fasting and how to go about it. Essential tips to make water fasting easy as well as how to have a smooth water fast have all been discussed.

In addition to fasting and exercise, what else can you do to have a smooth transition to autophagy?

This manual discussed many practices that can help you activate autophagy without stress. In addition to that, we have also discussed foods and supplements to eat to foster autophagy. These are food items that you can easily get at the grocery store.

You also need to be careful of some mistakes in your journey to activating autophagy so that you do not end up frustrated. We have examined a number of mistakes that people could innocently make. Knowledge of these mistakes will keep you on the right path and ensure you do the right thing.

All in all, autophagy is a potent phenomenon that can turn your life around. You can get a hold of your health and live a long, good life. You can age healthily without being subjected to devastating health issues like Alzheimer's disease, Parkinson's disease, dementia, and decreased cognitive function that comes with old age. You can be active and full of life.

I believe strict adherence to the teachings of this manual will be of immense help in allowing you to take back your health and well-being.

It is not only about reading and knowledge. Be sure to apply the teachings of this manual. For it is when you do that you are guaranteed to reap the health benefits of this age long phenomenon – autophagy!

References

1. Aihara, T (2016). Cold Shock as a Possible Remedy for Neurodegenerative Disease. Retrieved from https://clinmedjournals.org/articles/ijnn/international-journal-of-neurology-and-neurotherapy-ijnn-3-053.pdf

2. Better Health (2018). The 12 Important Benefits Of Autophagy. Retrieved from https://www.naomiwhittel.com/the-12-important-benefits-of-autophagy/

3. Bhatia, T. (2017). Water fasting has become super trendy, but is it powerfully healing – or really dangerous? Retrieved from https://www.mindbodygreen.com/articles/is-water-fasting-safe-or-healthy

4. Bhukel, A (2017) Spermidine boosts autophagy to protect from synapse aging. Retrieved from https://www.ncbi.nlm.nih.gov/pmc/articles/PMC5324840/

5. Dokladny, K (2015) Heat shock response and autophagy—cooperation and control. Retrieved from https://www.ncbi.nlm.nih.gov/pmc/articles/PMC4502786/

6. Group, E. (2017). The Health Benefits of Water Fasting. Retrieved from https://www.globalhealingcenter.com/natural-health/health-benefits-of-water-fasting/

7. Fallis J, (2018) 31 Powerful Ways to Induce Autophagy in the Brain. Retrieved from https://www.optimallivingdynamics.com/blog/31-powerful-ways-to-induce-autophagy-in-the-brain

8. Hd, G (2016) Electroacupuncture improves memory and protects neurons by regulation of the autophagy pathway in a rat model of Alzheimer's disease. Retrieved from https://www.ncbi.nlm.nih.gov/pubmed/26895770

9. Jockers, (2019) Water Fasting: 12 Strategies to Prepare Properly, Retrieved from https://drjockers.com/water-fasting/

10. Kondratova, A. (2012) Circadian clock and pathology of the ageing brain. Retrieved from https://www.ncbi.nlm.nih.gov/pmc/articles/PMC3718301/

11. Kim, H (2018). Autophagy in Human Skin Fibroblasts: Impact of Age. Retrieved from https://www.ncbi.nlm.nih.gov/pmc/articles/PMC6121946/

12. Kim HS, (2018). Autophagy in Human Skin Fibroblasts: Impact of Age. Retrieved from https://www.ncbi.nlm.nih.gov/pubmed/30071626

13. Land, S. (2019). How Long Until Autophagy Kicks In. Retrieved from https://siimland.com/how-long-until-autophagy-kicks-in/

14. Land, S. (2019). What's the Optimal Amount of Autophagy and Fasting? Retrieved from https://www.siimland.com/whats-the-optimal-amount-of-autophagy-and-fasting/

15. Land, S. (2019). 8 ways to get to autophagy faster. Retrieved from https://www.siimland.com/8-ways-to-get-into-autophagy-faster/

16. Land, S. (2019). Mistruths and Lies About Autophagy. Retrieved from https://www.siimland.com/mistruths-and-lies-about-autophagy/

17. Lark Ellen Farm, (2019) Pros and cons of water fasting. Retrieved from https://www.larkellenfarm.com/blogs/news/pros-and-cons-of-water-fasting

18. Land, S. (2019).. Negative Side effects of autophagy. Retrieved from https://siimland.com/negative-side-effects-of-autophagy/

19. Liu, Y (2017) Hyperbaric oxygen treatment attenuates neuropathic pain by elevating autophagy flux via inhibiting mTOR pathway. Retrieved from https://www.ncbi.nlm.nih.gov/pmc/articles/PMC5446542/

20. Luan, Y (2018) Chronic Caffeine Treatment Protects Against α-Synucleinopathy by Reestablishing Autophagy Activity in the Mouse Striatum. Retrieved from https://www.frontiersin.org/articles/336493

21. Maroon, J (2018) Review of the neurological benefits of phytocannabinoids. Retrieved from https://www.ncbi.nlm.nih.gov/pmc/articles/PMC5938896/

22. Pearson, K. (2017). How Omega-3 Fish Oil Affects Your Brain and Mental Health. Retrieved from https://www.healthline.com/nutrition/omega-3-fish-oil-for-brain-health

23. Pietrocola, F (2014) Coffee induces autophagy in vivo. Retrieved from https://www.ncbi.nlm.nih.gov/pmc/articles/PMC4111762/

24. Rosario-Acevedo, R (2013). Ganoderma lucidum (Reishi) induces autophagy in inflammatory breast cancer cells to promote cell death. Retrieved from http://cancerres.aacrjournals.org/content/73/8_Supplement/1672

25. Somma C, (2017) Vitamin D and Neurological Diseases: An Endocrine View. Retrieved from https://www.ncbi.nlm.nih.gov/pmc/articles/PMC5713448/

26. Sun, Y (2018) Sulforaphane Protects against Brain Diseases: Roles of Cytoprotective Enzymes. Retrieved from https://www.ncbi.nlm.nih.gov/pmc/articles/PMC5880051/

27. Tian, T (2016) Acupuncture promotes mTOR-independent autophagic clearance of aggregation-prone proteins in mouse brain. Retrieved from https://www.ncbi.nlm.nih.gov/pmc/articles/PMC4726430/

28. Toxnet, (2018) ACETYL-L-CARNITINE, Human Health Effects. Retrieved from https://toxnet.nlm.nih.gov/cgi-bin/sis/search/a?dbs+hsdb:@term+@DOCNO+7587

29. Wells K, (2019) Water Fasting Benefits, Dangers, & My Personal Experience. Retrieved from https://wellnessmama.com/345549/water-fasting/

30. Wu, S. (2011) Vitamin D, Vitamin D Receptor, and Macroautophagy in Inflammation and Infection. Retrieved from https://www.ncbi.nlm.nih.gov/pmc/articles/PMC3285235/

31. Zhang, Q. (2016) Pharmacologic preconditioning with berberine attenuating ischemia-induced apoptosis and promoting autophagy in neuron. Retrieved from https://www.ncbi.nlm.nih.gov/pmc/articles/PMC4846963/

Intermittent Fasting for Women

The COMPLETE Beginner's Guide to BURNING FAT, Heal Your BODY and Increase ENERGY through Keto Diet, Fasting and Autophagy. How to Do it Right and AVOID COMMON MISTAKES

Foreword

Whether we like it or not, obesity is a worldwide phenomenon which is spreading like wildfire amongst men and women all over the world, but especially in the Western world. There are a few factors which are known to boost obesity, like the food type consumed, the overall lifestyle and stress. Also, there are too many situations when obesity is not experienced just by itself, and it comes along with other diseases and medical conditions, like diabetes, heart, liver or kidney diseases and sometimes even cancer.

The food we eat is causing most of the health problems known to man these days, as it has plenty of carbohydrates and almost none other macronutrients. As it turns out, we can't live just on carbs, as we also need proteins, lipids (fats), and minerals and vitamins. Most of the food we consume today is processed, and I'm not referring just to fast food, I'm also referring to most of the food sold in supermarkets. If the food comes with a package and has very strange ingredients, then that food is processed. When checking the label for ingredients, you will also notice the nutritional value of it. Most of the processed food is very high in sugar or salt, while the protein or fat content is very low. That's why this kind of food has little to no nutritional value, yet it has too many calories. Therefore, processed food is more calorie dense than nutrient dense.

Sugar is a type of carbohydrate, which is very common in the food we eat. It's also one of the most harmful substances the human body can encounter. This substance is responsible for more deaths than drugs, alcohol or cigarettes. Governments have tried to make the consumers aware of the consequences of sugar consumption by marking the labels of processed food with different colors if the sugar level of the food or drink is above or normal compared to the daily recommended dosage. Some of them have even implemented a sugar tax imposed on soft drinks, juices or other products with very high levels of sugar.

Sugar contains glucose, which under most circumstances is the most used energy source for the body. However, energy is not produced by eating carbs, instead is generated by burning glucose. But this process only happens if the body engages in physical activity, and unfortunately eating carbs gets you more tired than energized. Just think about it! You consume plenty of carbs, so you have high levels of glucose. The glucose should be used by the body to generate energy, but this only happens when the body is active. If the glucose is not used, it will get stored in your blood, raising the insulin and high blood level. Sound familiar? This is how diabetes starts. However, processed food gives you a satiety feeling for a short period of time, so you will be craving more carbs from processed food in no time. More food means more calories and also more glucose. So not only will you be storing glucose, but you will also be storing fat, as you don't give the body the chance to burn calories and fat tissue. You are constantly feeding the body with this low-quality food, which requires higher levels of consumption. When you are eating that many calories, and you are not involved in physical activity, guess what? You will start to gain weight and unless you are changing what you eat and start to exercise, you will not be able to stop and reverse the weight gaining process.

Cutting down on carbs is the right solution when it comes to nutrition. But what exactly you can eat instead? The answer is simple. Try to replace them with healthy fats. As you change the energy source of your body, from glucose to fats, the body will start using fats, therefore burning them. This is how you can set the body to run on fats and to

117

decrease the fat tissue, thus reversing not only obesity, but also some other diseases and medical conditions as well.

Physical activity is what triggers the fat burning process if all the available glucose is burned and the body is using a different type of fuel, which can be found in the fat tissue, but also in high-fat meals. If we analyze the modern lifestyle, we can notice that there is little time to eat and even less time to exercise, as the modern job requires plenty of tasks to be done during the day and tight deadlines. This means more hours spent at work, less time to eat well and work out, and even less time to sleep. It also comes with plenty of stress. Remember, stress is a psychological condition which favors the consumption of processed food and snacks, so more calories. Therefore, it's fair to say that stress encourages obesity.

Women are more and more preoccupied with their looks, so being overweight is definitely something that can bother them. They are more keen on watching their weight than men, however, they are willing to spend less time exercising. Instead, women like to focus on trying all kinds of diets, many of them that are too radical and have harmful effects on their health. Trying diets without consulting a physician or a nutritionist has become a popular trend. Plenty of these diets require more or fewer restrictions, some of them are very harsh and most people break them because they can't stick to them anymore, or they are not feeling very well after trying them. After quitting the diet, most people will return to normal eating habits and will start to regain weight quite fast. Therefore, women should look for the best-balanced diets and should stick to them for a very long time, transforming them into a lifestyle. This book can show you a few very healthy alternatives when it comes to losing weight.

Chapter 1:

What Is Intermittent Fasting?

Nowadays, people are more and more exposed to processed foods, so there are higher chances of consuming a higher level of carbs (and therefore glucose). Since there are around 70% of the diseases known to man caused by processed food, people are trying to find a solution to this problem. Analyzing the eating habits of prehistoric humans, and even those from more recent ages, scientists have come with a solution, which was already implemented by some religious sects. This solution is called fasting, a very popular practice in religions like Islam, Judaism or even Christianity. The "pure" way to fast is to deprive yourself of food and water, with the intent of purifying your soul.

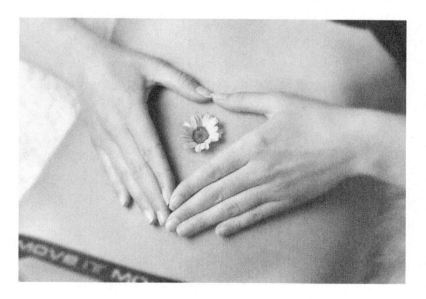

From a non-religious approach, fasting means the complete deprivation of food for a limited amount of time. Bearing this in mind, intermittent fasting (or IF for short) is an alternate cycle between feeding period and fasting period. There is no mention of what food you need to eat, so this procedure is more about scheduling your meals than what your meals include. The only thing you need to worry about is to sticking to the schedule. However, this doesn't mean that you can only eat fast food, or copious amounts of processed food, as one of the most important goals of this practice is to train your body to run on fats, not on glucose, and to favor the fat burning process. So, cutting down on carbs may be something very helpful when it comes to this diet.

Fasting doesn't mean the period between your meals of the day, as a period of 4 hours between meals is not considered fasting. Specialists would probably argue about what is the minimum period of time for fasting. Some would say between 12 and 14 hours, others would say at least 16 hours. However, when it comes to IF, you need to distinguish the difference between the fasting period and the fasted state. The first one is the period during which you are not consuming any calories at all, so you are not eating. The second term is more about a metabolic state during which the body starts to run on fats. The fasted state starts 12 hours after your last meal, after the glucose has been burned or processed, and the body can't seem to find other "fuel types" to use as energy. Switching to fats seems to be the obvious choice since glucose is no longer available. The energy from the fat tissue can only be released through the actions of ketones, molecules released by your liver specially designed to break through the fat cells. However, more details regarding ketones, ketosis and the keto-adaptation process can be found in the following chapters of this book.

Getting back to intermittent fasting, it's important to understand that the source of inspiration for it comes from history. Let's think about prehistoric humans and their lifestyle. In order to feed, these humans had to hunt, fish or pick fruits. Food wasn't always available, and nobody knew exactly when the next meal was planned to be. People were able to go for days without food. As a result, the prehistoric human was a lot stronger, faster and more agile than the modern-day human. Let's face it, the quality of food was a lot better back then, as everything was a natural (unlike today). However, as it turns out, fasting for a longer period can improve your concentration and can also increase the level of growth hormone. Therefore, fasting was not only very good for their muscle mass, but also for their focus. A more detailed approach on the benefits (and also the downsides) of intermittent fasting can be found in the chapter below. Food was not very available back then, and it required skill to procure it. Although it wasn't their intent, people were fasting on a regular basis back in the day. Having 3 meals each day was not possible, so they had a very different lifestyle than the one we have today. It was also a lot more active, as it involved running, climbing trees and possibly swimming, activities which are done today only by a few of us.

Some nutritionists would agree that intermittent fasting "is perhaps the oldest and most powerful dietary intervention imaginable."[1] IF is more about self-discipline, and less about starvation. If you "play your cards right", then your body will be able to resist starvation and you can go on fasting for a longer period. Control makes a difference in this case. Starvation may be caused by not having anything to eat (no control), whilst fasting is, in fact, a voluntary deprivation from food for different reasons, whether it's fat loss, overall health, or spiritual reasons. The

---

1 Fung, Jason, and Andreas Eenfeldt. "Intermittent Fasting for Beginners – The Complete Guide – Diet Doctor." *Diet Doctor*, 21 May 2019, www.dietdoctor.com/intermittent-fasting/.

purists would say that there is only one type of fast, the water fast. This is the most radical way of fasting, but there are also other ways, which are less harsh, and you will find more details about them in another chapter of this book.

Women are more sensitive when it comes to changes in their meal plan and the food they eat, but they should know that intermittent fasting is simply not for everyone. If they are breastfeeding, pregnant or underweight (also if they have an eating disorder such as anorexia), they shouldn't practice this way of eating. However, if they don't have any of these conditions, they are eligible for intermittent fasting, but still, they need to see a physician or a nutritionist first. If you are expecting unbelievable weight loss, then you will be most likely disappointed. This process is more about preparing the body for weight loss (in this case, fat burning) because it needs to be paired with physical exercise in order to be more effective.

It's said that intermittent fasting has 5 or 6 different stages, as seen below:

1) Ketosis - a metabolic state which should get activated 12 hours after your last meal. Ketone level is going up, and this favors the breaking down of fat tissue, thus releasing the energy stored in the fat cells. Let's say that you have the last meal at 6 pm, this means you should be entering the ketosis phase the next day at 6 am. The human brain is capable of using 60% of the glucose whilst the body

rests.[2] Ketones are starting to become the default fuel type for now.

2) Fat-burning mode - 18 hours after your last meal, the body runs now just on fats, as the ketones level is very high, so more ketones mean more fats burned.

3) Recycling old cells' components - a state which occurs 24 hours after your last meal. Not only these parts are being recycled, but also other misfolded or old proteins are being destroyed. These proteins can be associated with diseases like Parkinson and Alzheimer's. This phase is also known as *autophagy*.

4) The growth hormone level reaches a level which is 5 times higher than the one at the beginning of your fast. This happens after 48 hours of the fasting period, during which you didn't have any calories at all. This hormone is responsible for preserving your muscle mass but also can prevent fat tissue accumulation.

5) After 54 hours of fasting, the insulin level reaches unbelievably low levels. The lower your insulin level is, the more active it gets. Apparently, the best way to activate your insulin and let it determine how to do its job (regulating the blood sugar level, or lowering it) is to lower it. Well, this is what intermittent fasting does to the insulin level.

6) Recycling old immune cells and generating brand new ones. This phase happens after 72 hours of fasting.

---

2 Jarreau, Paige, and Essential Information. "The 5 Stages of Intermittent Fasting." *LIFE Apps | LIVE and LEARN*, 26 Feb. 2019, lifeapps.io/fasting/the-5-stages-of-intermittent-fasting/.

Chapter 2:
Benefits and Side Effects of
Intermittent Fasting

There are plenty of diets out there, all promising you the impossible. Incredible weight loss, with no mention of any side effects. You are probably fed up with the "lose x pounds in 30 days, guaranteed" approach. Many of these diets are not backed up by science, or in other words, there is not any scientific research to prove these diets actually deliver what they promise. They focus only on the weight loss process, suggesting meal plans that are extremely radical in some cases.

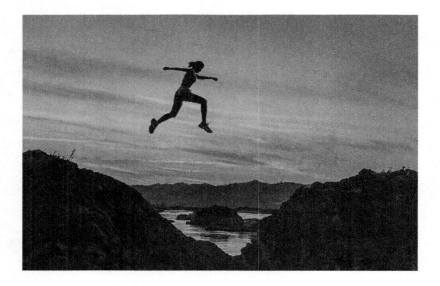

Diets mean nutrient deprivation in most cases, but they are plenty of cases when these diets have harmful effects on your health. Unlike other diets, focused on the weight loss process in an incredibly short amount of time, intermittent fasting is focusing more on your health, as nutritionists believe that health should be the most important factor, and only a healthy body can have a long and sustainable weight loss process. Unlike the other diets, which have a "hit and run" approach, IF is something for the long run and should be regarded as a way of life, not like a meal plan to be implemented for a few weeks. By checking out the benefits below, you can better understand why this process is so beneficial for your body.

The main benefits of intermittent fasting can be summarized in 8 points:

- eliminates precancerous and cancerous cells
- shifts easily into nutritional ketosis
- reduces the fat tissue
- enhances the gene expression for health span and longevity
- induces autophagy and the apoptotic cellular repair or cleaning
- improves your insulin sensitivity
- reduces inflammation and oxidative stress
- increases neuroprotection and cognitive effects

To expand on the benefits of this practice, intermittent fasting can have positive impacts over the fat loss process, disease prevention, anti-aging, therapeutic benefits (psychological, spiritual and physical), mental performance, physical fitness (improved metabolism, wind, and endurance, the great effect over bodybuilding).

Intermittent Fasting for the Weight Loss Process

As you restrain yourself from eating, the body will no longer have available glucose to use in order to produce energy. Therefore, it will use ketones to break the fat tissue open and release the energy stored in there. This is how the body will burn your existing fat in order to generate energy. When it comes to diets, they are not designed for the long run, and as soon as you break the diet, you will start gaining weight again. Intermittent fasting is something that you can try for a lifetime because it is easy to stick to it, and it doesn't involve any special meal plan. So, you can still eat your favorite foods, as long as you schedule your meals, allowing a smaller eating window and a longer fasting period. IF induces ketosis and eventually autophagy, which will definitely mean reducing the fat reserves.

Intermittent Fasting for Preventing Diseases

What if you found out that intermittent fasting is, in fact, a cure for several different diseases and medical conditions? You would definitely become more interested in this process. There are a few studies that show the beneficial effects IF has on your health. A study published in the *World Journal of Diabetes* has shown that patients with type 2 diabetes on short-term daily intermittent fasting experience a lower body weight, but also a better variability of post-meal glucose.

Other benefits this diet has are:

- enhances the markers of stress resistance
- reduces the blood pressure and inflammation
- better lipid levels and glucose circulation, which may lead to a lower risk of cardiovascular disease, neurological diseases like Parkinson's and Alzheimer's, and also cancer

Intermittent Fasting for the Anti-Aging Process

The modern-day lifestyle includes too much stress and is too sedentary. Whether we like it or not, these factors have a great contribution to the aging process. You are probably wondering what intermittent fasting can do the slow down this process, as we all know that it can't be stopped. IF is not "the fountain of youth" and it will not grant you immortality, but it can still lower the blood pressure and reduce oxidative damage, enhance your insulin sensitivity and reduce your fat mass. Coincidence or not, all of these are factors are known to improve your health and longevity. Intermittent fasting is one of the triggering factors of autophagy, a process known for destroying and replacing old cell parts with new ones, at any level within your body. Such a process can slow down the aging process.

Intermittent Fasting Practiced for Therapeutic Benefits

When it comes to therapeutic benefits, the most important ones are physical, spiritual and psychological. In terms of **physical benefits**, intermittent fasting is a powerful cure for diabetes, but it can also prove to be very useful for reducing seizure-related brain damage and seizures themselves, but also for improving the symptoms of arthritis. This practice also has a spiritual value, as it's widely practiced for religious purposes across the globe. Although fasting is regarded as penance by some practitioners, it's also a practice for purifying your body and soul (according to the religious approach).

Intermittent fasting is also about exercising control and will, over your body and your feelings. Achieving absolute control over your power and mind is a very powerful **psychological** benefit. You can ignore hunger, restrain yourself from eating for a certain period of time. In other words, IF is also associated with mind training and can also improve your self-esteem. A successful intermittent fasting regime can have very powerful effects from a psychological point of view. A study has shown that women practicing IF had amazing results in terms of senses of control, reward, pride, and achievement.

Intermittent Fasting for Better Mental Performance

IF also enhances the cognitive function and also is very useful when it comes to boosting your brain power. There are several factors of intermittent fasting which can support this claim. First of all, it boosts the level of brain-derived neurotrophic factor (also known as BDNF), which is a protein in your brain that can interact with the parts of your brain responsible for controlling cognitive and memory functions as well as learning. BDNF can even protect and stimulate the growth of new brain cells. Through IF, you will enter the ketogenic state, during which your body turn fat into energy, by using ketones. Ketones can also feed your brain, and therefore improve your mental acuity, productivity, and energy.

Intermittent Fasting for an Improved Physical Fitness

This process influences not only your brain but also your digestive system. By setting a small feeding window and a larger fasting period, you will encourage the proper digestion of food. This leads to a proportional and healthy daily intake of food and calories. The more you get used to this process, the less you will experience hunger. If you are worried about slowing your metabolism, think again! IF *enhances* your metabolism, it makes metabolism more flexible, as the body has now the capability to run on glucose or fats for energy, in a very effective way. In other words, intermittent fasting leads to better metabolism.

Oxygen use during exercise is a crucial part of the success of your training. You simply can't have performance without adjusting your breathing habits during workouts. VO2 max represents the maximum amount of oxygen your body can use per minute or per kilogram of body weight. In popular terms, VO2 max is also referred to as "wind".

The more oxygen you use, the better you will be able to perform. Top athletes can have twice the VO2 level of those without any training. A study focused on the VO2 levels of a fasted group (they just skipped breakfast) and a non-fasted group (they had breakfast an hour before). For both groups, the VO2 level was at 3.5 L/min at the beginning, and after the study, the level showed a significant increase of "wind" for the fasting group (9.7%), compared to just 2.5% increase in the case of those with breakfast.

Intermittent Fasting for Bodybuilding

Having a narrow feeding window automatically mean fewer meals, so you can concentrate the daily calorie intake into just 1-2 consistent meals. Bodybuilders find this approach a lot more pleasing than having the same calorie consumption split into 5 or 6 different meals throughout the day. It's said that you need a specific amount of proteins just to maintain your muscle mass. However, muscle mass can be also maintained through intermittent fasting, a process which doesn't focus specifically on protein intake. Remember, the growth hormone reaches unbelievable levels after 48 hours of fasting, so you can easily maintain your muscles without eating many proteins, or having protein bars or shakes.

As you already know, nothing is perfect and intermittent fasting is no exception. There are a few **side effects** that you need to worry about, like:

- **hunger** is perhaps the most common side effect of this way of eating, but the more you get used to IF, the less hunger you will feel

- beware of **constipation,** as when you eat less, you will not have to go to the toilet very often, so you can feel constipated at the beginning
- **headaches** should be expected when fasting. Food deprivation is a direct cause of these headaches. However, controlling your hunger and getting used to fasting, will be the best weapon to fight against these headaches
- during intermittent fasting, you might experience muscle cramps, heartburn, and dizziness
- in the case of athletic women, or those with very low body fat percentage, intermittent fasting may lead to a higher risk of irregular periods and lower chances of conception (so it reduces fertility for these women)

Chapter 3:

Types of Intermittent Fasting

There are several intermittent fasting programs you can choose from according to your needs and goals you want to achieve. Burning fats seems to be one of the main goals of IF, regardless of the program you choose.

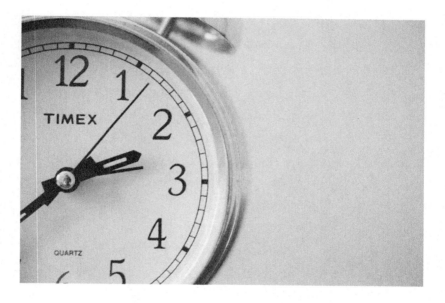

Considering the fasting period you are trying to set, or the reduction of calories, there are a few fasting programs which are worth to be mentioned.

1) **The Leangains Program** (also known as the 16/8 hours fast) is a daily fasting program which allows the body plenty of time to burn fats. It splits the day into 2 periods: 8 hours of feeding and 16 hours of fasting. The 16/8 hours fast program is a program which can be easily practiced by most of the women out there,

unless they have a special medical condition or they are pregnant, trying to conceive a baby or have an eating disorder. It usually involves skipping one important meal of the day, and most nutritionists would suggest skipping breakfast. Considering breakfast the most important meal of the day is a myth, as in this case, you can easily skip breakfast and let your body burn fats. Scientists believe that the body goes into the fasted state 12 hours after your last meal. In this state, glucose is no longer available, so the body will start to run on fats. It's the perfect time to exercise. If you have the last meal at 6 pm, then you will start the fasted state at 6 am the next day. You can choose several options for physical exercise, and if it's more intense than it's even better. Jogging, cycling, swimming, or intense gym training are perfect options for morning exercise which are guaranteed to burn fat. The 16 hour fasting period should be respected, and you shouldn't consume any calories during this period. Plus, at least 7 hours during this fasting period you should be asleep. The Leangains program involves setting up a few things like:

- when to start your feeding window, and how long should it last? Although the recommended time frame for the eating period is 8 hours, you can even go lower than that, for example having an eating period of 6 hours (the lower your feeding window is, the better for your body). You can start it at 10 am and finish it at 6 pm.

- the fasting period is very important, as it needs to be around 16 hours or more, and it should include your sleeping period as well. During these 16 hours, you need to avoid consuming any kind of calories, so you can only drink water.

- don't forget about physical exercise, as you need to establish when it's the best time to work out. All specialists would agree that intense training during the fasted state (more than 12 hours after your last meal) is the perfect time to work out, as your body will use only fats to generate energy.

Following this program is not an easy thing to do, in fact, it can be a bit of a challenge. However, to make sure you have very good results when implementing the Leangains program, make sure you respect the following tips:

- Make sure you consume enough proteins in the feeding window but don't try to compensate in one day if you had several days with lower protein intake.
- Working out is a must for this program.
- If you plan on consuming carbs, make sure you do it on the workout days, as you definitely want to burn the excess glucose.
- Focus on eating consistent meals (by consistent I mean nutrient-dense food, not calorie bombs with very low nutritional value) during the feeding period, and make sure you don't consume any calories during the fasting period (drink only water, don't eat anything, not even snacks).
- Since physical exercise is a part of this program, make sure you don't eat anything before the training, and have the most consistent meal of the day right after training.
- If you don't have any exercise planned for a specific day, you still need to have the first meal as the most consistent one of the day.

Whether you choose to have a feeding window of 6 or 8 hours is up to you. It's possible to squeeze all 3 main meals of the day in 8 hours, but in 6 hours it's impossible. Having a daily fasting process is very good for your body, as it can function at optimal parameters and also burn fat while doing it. This program is highly appreciated by bodybuilders. Although there is no mention of what kind of food you need to consume on a daily basis, it's recommended to cut down on carbs to make the program more effective. Lowering the eating window to just 4 hours per day takes intermittent fasting to a whole different level, called The Warrior Diet, but this program is too radical to be implemented by most women practically.

2) **The 24 hours fast,** or also known as *Eat Stop Eat,* is a program promoted by Brad Pilon, a fitness enthusiast. It means literally fasting for 24 hours, so no eating or snacking at all during this period. Just water. During this day you will allow plenty of time for the body to burn fats and experience all the other benefits of intermittent fasting. Therefore, you can have a normal feeding day, followed by 24 hours of fasting. If you have your last meal on Tuesday at 6pm, this means that you will have the next meal on Wednesday at 6pm. For better results, you can also work out on the fasting day and you can alternate the feeding days with fasting days for 2 or 3 times during any given week, depending on what you are trying to achieve. Not consuming anything in the fasting window doesn't mean you will have to compensate the calories in the feeding window. So make sure you don't overdo it when it comes to eating. Fasting for 24 hours or more shouldn't be a very tough practice, as in some religions fasting is a normal habit practiced widely. So if religious people can do it, so can you. Healthy food and physical exercise are also highly recommended, although this program doesn't mention anything about the food you will need to eat or what kind of exercise you need to practice. Nutritionists recommend the day-long fast at least once a few weeks, however, there is nothing wrong with trying it on a more regular basis.

The more often you use this type of fast, the more spectacular will be the results.

3) **The Alternate Day Fast (also known as 36/12 hour fast)** is a perfect example of fasting for a longer period, and unlike other intermittent fasting programs, this one was actually developed by a doctor, so this program can get extra credit for this specific reason. A famous nutritionist, Dr. James B. Johnson, is the person responsible for developing the Alternate Day Fast, as he wrote a book dedicated to this program, called "The Alternate Day Diet." The 36/12 hour fast involves having a 12-hour feeding period (which is quite normal, you can have all 3 main meals of the day during this feeding window), followed by 36 hours of fasting. It may sound long, but this fasting period is totally doable. However, to make sure the fasting period is easier to endure, make sure you have proper nutrient-dense food during the feeding period. Healthy fats and protein intake should be higher than the carb consumption. Since this program was not developed by a bodybuilder, it doesn't mention anywhere that you need to work out, however, to have better results you really should. This method is not that strict, as you can easily eat whatever you like (as long as it's healthy) in the 12 hour eating window, and that's why it should be perfect for beginners.

You will need to follow a few simple rules like:

a) Make sure you fast for at least 36 hours
b) Eat normally during the 12 hours feeding period
c) Although you can eat anything you want, it's highly recommended to have nutrient-dense foods instead of calorie-dense ones

During this program, you will need to establish the feeding and fasting windows:

1) Establish your feeding period as 12 hours during a day. Let's say you have your first meal at 7 am and the last one at 7 pm on a Monday, so you can repeat the same feeding schedule 4 days during a week (Monday, Wednesday, Friday, Sunday);
2) Your fasting window is 36 hours and should start after the last meal. Therefore, in this case, it should start at 7 pm on Monday and should last until 7 am on Wednesday.

This program was already tested on people, and it delivered really interesting results. The Alternate Day Diet not only has effects on the weight loss process, but it also has effects on your health. Volunteers who tested this program "lost on average 8% of their body weight over an eight-week period and experienced benefits such as reduced inflammation improved insulin resistance and better cellular energy production".[3] It's no surprise that intermittent fasting programs are capable of lowering blood pressure and this one makes no exception. It can also be the right program to induce autophagy and to ease arthritis. Having 36 hours of "pure" fast can be a bit too radical, especially for women, that's why Dr. James B. Johnson considers that you can have a very small calorie intake in the fasting period, around 500 calories. The rule, in this case, would be to consume 20% of the normal calorie intake. That's why, from his point of view, feeding days are considered Up Days, whilst the fasting days are considered Down Days. The 20% rule in the Down Days can apply in the first 2 weeks, but from week 3 you can increase the calorie intake from 20% to 35%. You are probably wondering what are you allowed to consume during the Down Days, and fruits and smoothies are the right choices. In

---

3 Matus, Mizpah. *Alternate Day Diet*, www.freedieting.com/alternate-day-diet.

order to make the program more efficient, you will also have to eat healthy during the eating window. Therefore, eating keto or Mediterranean is the right thing to do. Food types or drinks like chicken, fish, turkey, fruits, vegetables, eggs white, oats, whole wheat bread, high-fiber cereal, pasta, Shirataki noodles, and red wine should definitely be in your diet. Working out can't do you any harm, even on the fasting days, so you can combine this program with training for better fat-burning results.

The Alternate Day Fast has plenty of advantages like:

- it doesn't come with restrictions in terms of food, however, it's highly recommended to eat healthily and include the food types mentioned above in your diet
- the method is simple enough and easy to follow it for a long period of time
- deprivation is not something you need to worry about, as you can eat whatever you like during the feeding period
- you can trust this program even more, as it was developed by a real doctor
- it looks like this method can improve conditions like asthma
- this method can improve the metabolism and extend the lifespan (just like any other intermittent fasting method)

However, there are some downsides to this method, as you can see below:

- there is a higher risk of experiencing fatigue, dizziness, and hunger in the first days of practicing this program

- the method as developed by Dr. James B. Johnson doesn't mention anything about physical exercise, probably just to point out the major role the program has in the fat-burning process
- if you have an eating disorder like anorexia, you definitely shouldn't try this program

The Alternate Day Fast allows you to consume calories in the fasting days, and it doesn't mention any training or working out during this program. However, this doesn't mean that it's forbidden to practice a bit of physical exercise. Some people may consider this program the easiest one out there, so perhaps when they are thinking about trying intermittent fasting, this can be the first program they can try. However, if you are pregnant, breastfeeding, or have an eating disorder, you may need to stay away from IF.

4) **Water Fasting** is the "purest" program when it comes to intermittent fasting, and it's also the most radical one. No matter how healthy you are, you shouldn't try this program without the support and supervision of a physician. This should be tried as a last resort if no other IF programs work, or if you want to achieve faster results. Even though people can go for hundreds of days using just water, probably the perfect example is one of an obese man who managed to fast for 382 days (consuming just water and vitamins) and lose 276 pounds. You will need to keep in mind that this method deprives you of all nutrients, minerals, and vitamins that come from food, so you better have a really strong reason to try it. Water fasting is regarded as a very good program for detoxing and fat burning. It will definitely make your body switch to the metabolic state of ketosis, and then it will induce autophagy (more about autophagy in a future chapter). This program is definitely not for everyone, as it's the best example of fasting for a longer period. Having nothing to eat for several days

(people might even try it more than a week) is not very comfortable. You will experience all the possible side effects of intermittent fasting with this program like fatigue, dizziness, and hunger, but you will maximize the benefits of fat burning, disease prevention and other benefits to your health and physical condition. Of course, the method doesn't mention any workout or any sort of training. You should only try working out if you feel up to it, as when you are not having anything to eat at all, you will lack the necessary nutrients and you will not have glucose or fat from which the body can extract the energy. The second day of water fasting is probably the hardest one, as you will feel most hungry during this day. It's important to set your mind and overcome this situation and move on with the fasting process. As long as the days go by, you will feel more comfortable fasting. It's also important to keep your mind occupied, and not to think about food. However, you don't have to exaggerate and fast for too many days. You should fast for as long as you feel capable, but only with the supervision of a physician. There is also an alternative to the water fast, which is a bit less radical. It's called juice or broth fasting. Whilst juice can have plenty of vitamins and is mostly made out of fruits, you should try juices made out of vegetables because fruits have a lot more sugar than veggies. The broth is a type of soup which can have some proteins and nutrients, and you can also put a bit of fat into it. The human body can last for a few days without water, and for plenty more days without food. However, too many days without food is definitely not something recommendable. That's why most doctors would not recommend water fasting for more than 72 hours. If you are thinking about trying intermittent fasting, then you definitely need to start with a method which is a lot easier, like the ones mentioned previously in this chapter. Fasting for a very long time doesn't necessarily mean that it will bring you better results than if you fast for 16, 20 or 24 hours.

In terms of fat burning, you can have better results with trying the Leangains Program associated with intense training and healthy food (keto diet seems to be the best choice).

5) **Fast Mimicking or Fat Fasting** is a very interesting alternative fasting program. What if you can actually eat and still fast? This is the best question to ask yourself when you are thinking of trying this program. Intermittent fasting is a procedure designed to make your body run on fats, and therefore burn more fats. Let's face it, water fasting is not for everyone, just for a few. Other fasting programs may be already too harsh in terms of lowering the feeding window and expanding the fasting window, so you will spend more time in the fasting window, not eating anything. The worst part is that the fasting window is not limited to sleeping. There is actually a method of fasting which doesn't involve splitting your day into fasting and feeding windows, so you don't have to worry about that. You can consume fats (yes, that's correct) in order to lose weight. You are probably asking, how is this possible? The answer is very simple.

"Your body doesn't distinguish dietary fat from metabolizing dietary fat, and therefore remains in the fasted state. This gives you the benefits of fasting while allowing you the macro and micronutrients your body needs to get into ketosis and all the benefits from brain and body fueled by ketones".[4]

Sound interesting enough? Well, take a look below to find out more about the advantages and benefits:

---

4 The A-Z of Intermittent Fasting: Everything You Need to Know. (n.d.). *Perfect Keto*, p. 18.

- it improves and regenerates the immune system
- it suppresses the precancerous and cancerous cells
- it triggers autophagy
- it activates ketosis which will help with the fat burning process
- it lowers the C-reactive protein and the oxidative stress
- it enhances your gene expression, and therefore it increases your longevity
- it can help improve your healthy stem cells, regenerative markers and fasting glucose
- it boosts your mental performance and also BDNF (brain-derived neurotrophic factor), which is crucial for the survival and growth of the new brain neurons

Chapter 4:

The Weight Loss Process

Weight loss is one of the main benefits of intermittent fasting, regardless of the program you use. Everyone likes to lose some weight, especially if they are overweight, but do they want to lose muscle mass, or do they want to burn fat? Most would say that they want to burn fat, as fat is not aesthetically pleasing, and can also lead to health issues. However, if you are expecting miracles from any IF programs in terms of fat loss, think again! This lifestyle prepares the body to burn fats, but physical exercise is what enhances the fat burning process. Intermittent fasting is able to switch the default "fuel type" of the body from glucose to fat, so every activity that you do will break down the fat tissue and release the energy stored in there.

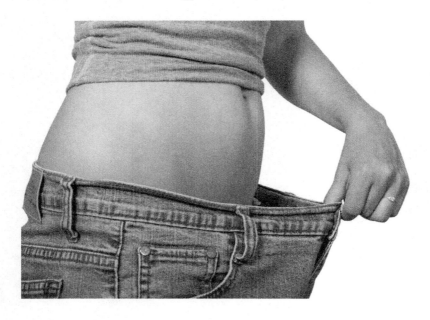

When it comes to the fat burning process, you really have to understand the term *ketosis*, which is a metabolic state during which the ketone body levels are going high and the insulin level is going low. Insulin is something that we are all aware of, but what about ketones? They are a class of organic compounds capable of breaking down the fat tissues in order to release the energy stored within them. A normal diet will get your body fed using glucose, which the body will need to burn in order to produce energy. Glucose can mostly be found in carbs, but they are also found in proteins. It's highly unlikely to burn all the glucose you consume, though, especially when the body is not engaged in physical activity. If the glucose is not consumed it gets stored in your blood and therefore it raises the blood sugar level. Not consuming carbs (rich in glucose), and even not consuming anything at all, will lower the insulin level and will raise the levels of ketones.

Through intermittent fasting, the body can enter ketosis 12 hours after your last meal. At this point, the body can't find any glucose available to use, so it's starting to look for alternative energy sources. The ketone bodies are multiplying, and they will help the body burn fat tissue to release the energy stored there.

If ketosis is a metabolic state during which the insulin, blood sugar and ketones bodies are all getting at an appropriate level, the keto-adaptation process is somewhat different, as it trains your body to run on ketones and fat as the default source of energy. So you don't have to rely on glucose as your energy source, you can instead use your existing stored fat or dietary fat (by dietary fat we mean the fats you eat through your meal plan, low-carb-high-fat [LCHF] diets are recommended). You can reach the keto-adaptation process through intermittent fasting when your body will use the energy stored in your fat reserves, but you can also induce it through nutritional ketosis (the keto diet is what can get you in this phase). "To become keto-adapted, you have to go through a period of being in ketosis where your liver's enzymes and metabolic processes change so you could have the ability to burn fat for fuel, but it's not necessary to be in ketosis all the time to maintain keto adaptation. You can briefly dip in and out of the ketosis for a day or two without fully losing it."[5]

Intermittent fasting is a process that can help you lose weight, mostly in terms of fat, but it doesn't mean that it will work miracles on you. It's not the kind of program to promise you will lose 10-20 pounds per week. Any diet promising you this is either unhealthy or just lying to get you on board. IF is instead one of the healthiest and most sustainable ways to lose weight, as you can use this program for a very long time, while enjoying plenty of health benefits yourself, during which time you will slowly notice yourself losing some pounds. In the case of other diets, the more drastic the diet is, the more pounds you lose, but the more likely is for you to quit it soon and start gaining pounds immediately. Intermittent fasting is a program you can stick to, which encourage you to lose weight in a natural way. It's more of a lifestyle, which means that by following this way of eating you will not gain weight, but you will slowly lose weight, without having to cut out your favorite types of food.

Another very important aspect of IF is physical exercise, as it can make the difference between a very moderate weight loss (in terms of fat burn) and a very visible one. HIIT (High-Intensity Interval Training) can be the most effective for people to lose weight. It requires training very intensely with heavy weights and having just a few seconds as a break between exercises. By repeating the exercises, people feel their

---

5 Land, S. (2018). *Metabolic autophagy*. Independently Published, p. 285-286

body burn fat and gain tone. However, this is something that isn't suitable for all women, so cardio and endurance exercises are recommended for those who are not suited to HIIT. Don't let the body rest too much, because this is how you will be able to burn fats. Having just 30 seconds of break time between exercises may be the ideal way to work out. This applies if you are going to the gym, you can also try some other forms of physical exercises, like jogging and swimming, or even cycling. Doing some ab exercises, squats, pushups and other physical exercises which can be done from home is also highly recommended. Exercising during the fasting period may be the best way to burn fats, as you will force your body to activate the ketones and break down the fat tissue for some fats.

If you are consuming dietary fat, the body will first consume it first, and only then switch to your stored fat. The transition is more smoothly than having glucose and then switching to the fat reserves, as your ketones are already very active in this case and it will not take too much time to switch the "fuel type" from glucose to fat. You can compare your body to a car, and the fat your body uses as an energy source with "biofuel."

To sum up, intermittent fasting can prepare your body for the fat-burning process, but the real fat burn is happening through physical exercise. By setting your body to run on fats, this will maximize the effects of the fat-burning process through physical exercise, as every bit of energy comes from fat. That's why exercising and fasting practiced more frequently can have better results in terms of weight loss than just doing fasting alone. Remember, your body needs to be in a keto-adapted state in order to burn fats very efficiently, and intermittent fasting can help you achieve this state, but especially in combination with a keto diet. More details on the keto diet can be found in a future chapter.

145

Chapter 5:

Autophagy

The term autophagy can trace its roots to Ancient Greece and is the joining of two notions: "auto" (which means self) and "phagein" (which means to eat), therefore, in common words, autophagy means to eat oneself. A more detailed definition of this term can show us that is a mechanism used to get rid of old and damaged cell parts like cells membranes, organelles, and proteins. This can happen when the body lacks the energy to preserve the damaged and old cell machinery (which is composed of different cells parts mentioned above).

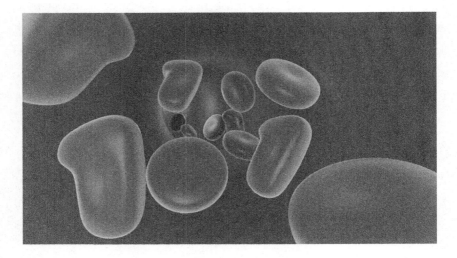

In other words, autophagy degrades and recycles all sorts of cellular parts, but it shouldn't be confused with apoptosis, which is the process of scheduling cell death. Although it sounds a bit cruel, apoptosis is exactly like an old car which is not working anymore, so you will need to dispose of the old and not-functioning parts. Apoptosis gets rid of the cells and replaces them with new ones. Autophagy basically does the same thing, but at a subcellular level.

The first autophagy studies were conducted on yeast, and the progress on this particular field of expertise also led to a Nobel Prize in October 2016. Dr. Yoshinori Ohsumi won the Nobel Prize in Physiology or Medicine for his "discoveries of the mechanisms for autophagy." However, autophagy is not present just in yeast, it's present in every living organism, even in the human body.

Since we already covered what autophagy is, you are probably wondering what can trigger it. "Autophagy, a cellular cleaning process, gets activated in response to certain types of metabolic stress, including nutrient deprivation, growth factor depletion, and hypoxia. Even without adequate circulation, each cell may break down subcellular parts and recycle those into new proteins or energy as required to survive"[6].

Although understanding this process may require a bit of studying and learning some terms which are quite complicated, you need to know that autophagy can be viewed as a cellular housekeeper, because of its main functions:

- to eliminate defective proteins and organelles
- to prevent the accumulation of abnormal protein aggregates
- to eliminate intracellular pathogens

_____

6 Fung, Jason. "Autophagy – a Cure for Many Present-Day Diseases?" *Diet Doctor*, 19 Dec. 2017, www.dietdoctor.com/autophagy-cure-many-present-day-diseases.

That sounds interesting, however, you are probably still asking yourself why you should force your body to do this process (as it has to be induced somehow). The list of benefits is very long, but you can see them all below:

- "Providing cells with molecular building blocks and energy
- Recycling damaged proteins, organelles, and aggregates
- Regulating functions of cells' mitochondria, which help produce energy but can be damaged by oxidative stress
- Clearing damaged endoplasmic reticulum and peroxisomes
- Protecting the nervous system and encouraging the growth of brain and nerve cells. Autophagy seems to improve cognitive function, brain structure, and neuroplasticity.
- Supporting the growth of heart cells and protecting against **heart disease**
- **Enhancing the immune system** by eliminating intracellular pathogens
- Defending against misfolded, toxic proteins that contribute to a number of amyloid diseases
- Protecting stability of DNA
- Preventing damage to healthy tissues and organs (known as necrosis)
- Potentially fighting cancer, neurodegenerative disease, or other illnesses"[7]

Now, this list sounds very convincing, especially since most of the benefits mentioned in it are backed up by research studies. You are

---

7 Levy, Jillian. "Benefits of Autophagy, Plus How to Induce It." *Dr. Axe*, 4 Sept. 2018, draxe.com/benefits-of-autophagy/.

probably wondering right now, how to induce autophagy and experience all its benefits. Specialists suggest that there are 3 ways to trigger the autophagy process.

"When does autophagy occur? Autophagy is active in all cells but is increased in response to stress or nutrient deprivation (fasting or starvation). This means you can utilize 'good stressors' like exercise and temporary calorie-restriction (fasting) to boost autophagic processes. Both of these strategies have been linked with benefits like weight control, longevity, and inhibition of many age-associated diseases."[8]

The first way to induce autophagy is through intermittent fasting. Restraining yourself from eating food for a while will eventually trigger autophagy. It's said that after 24 hours since your last meal, the autophagy process will start. This is probably the best way to induce autophagy, as it's a lifestyle habit that you completely control. Just like mentioned above, you will need to fast for a longer period in order to trigger autophagy. That's why it is recommended to use the Alternate Day Fast or Water Fasting in order to start autophagy. If you do choose the Alternate Day Fast, make sure you don't eat anything at all during the 36 hour fast, and make sure you don't consume any calories either. So try to stay away from juices or other soft drinks, as they are very high in sugar. If you do try the water fasting method, make sure you stick to it for at least 2 or 3 days, as the recommended fasting period, in this case, is 24 to 48 hours. For your own health and to induce autophagy, you should try the Alternate Day Fast, with no calories in the fasting window, or if you feel up to it, you can try the

---

8 Levy, Jillian. "Benefits of Autophagy, Plus How to Induce It." *Dr. Axe*, 4 Sept. 2018, draxe.com/benefits-of-autophagy/.

water fasting program for 2 to 3 days, once every 3 months. Just judging by the list of benefits this process has, I believe it's totally worth it to restrain yourself from eating for a period of 36, 48 or 72 hours.

The second way of triggering autophagy is the **ketogenic diet**. Although this type of diet will be detailed in a later chapter of this book, you still need to understand the basics of this meal plan (also known as the keto diet). The basic principle of this dietary plan is to cut down on carbs, therefore this diet suggests a low carb high fat intake. Basically, it suggests replacing the carbs with healthy fats, in order for the body to burn fat. How is this possible? Well, apparently once the body switches the primary fuel type from glucose to fat, it will just start to burn fat. It's up to you how much fat you consume in order for your body to burn more of your own fat reserves. The keto diet induces the metabolic state of ketosis, during which the ketone bodies are multiplying and the insulin level is decreasing. Once the insulin level gets low enough, the insulin will become active and will start to regulate (lower) the blood sugar level, and therefore decrease the risk of diabetes. Ketones are just some organic compounds produced by your liver capable of breaking down the fat tissue in order to release the energy stored therein. The keto-adaptation process is when your body runs on ketones and fats, whether we're talking dietary fat or fat tissue. Speaking of dietary fat, the keto diet requires 75% of your daily nutrient intake to be lipids, and just 5 to 10% to be carbs. The rest can be proteins. I know it sounds strange. How can you eat that much fat and still *burn* fat, and lose weight? The body simply won't notice the difference between your fat reserves and the ones you consume, so it will burn them nevertheless. Olive oil, coconut or almond oil should be something you consume a lot more often. Also, avocado, high-fat cheeses, nuts, seeds, and other types of vegetables should be consumed. More on the keto ingredients can be found in a later chapter of this book. "In response to such severe carb restriction, you'll begin to start producing ketone bodies that have many protective effects. Studies suggest that ketosis can also cause starvation-induced autophagy, which has neuroprotective functions. For example, in animal studies when rats are put on the ketogenic diet, the keto diet has been shown to start autophagic pathways that reduce brain injury during and after seizures."[9]

"Another 'good stress' that can induce autophagy is exercising. Recent research has shown that 'Exercise induces autophagy in multiple organs involved in metabolic regulation, such as muscle, liver, pancreas and adipose tissue. While exercise has many benefits, it's actually a form of stress because it breaks down tissues, causing them to be repaired and grow back stronger. It's not exactly clear yet how much exercise is needed to boost autophagy, but research does suggest that intense exercise is probably most beneficial. In skeletal and cardiac muscle tissue, as little as 30 minutes of exercise can be sufficient to induce autophagy.'"[10] Most people who try intermittent fasting are also able to work out, and once they get used to it, they will feel more energetic and will have the extra motivation to exercise and fast. If you combine all of them together, you should be able to induce autophagy even faster.

---

9 Levy, Jillian. "Benefits of Autophagy, Plus How to Induce It." *Dr. Axe*, 4 Sept. 2018, draxe.com/benefits-of-autophagy/.

10 Levy, Jillian. "Benefits of Autophagy, Plus How to Induce It." *Dr. Axe*, 4 Sept. 2018, draxe.com/benefits-of-autophagy/.

There are plenty of things to find out about autophagy, and you also need to know about its 3 main pathways:

1. " mTOR – sensitive to dietary protein
2. AMPK – 'reverse fuel gauge' of the cell
3. Insulin-sensitive to protein and carbohydrates

When these nutrient sensors detect low nutrient availability, they tell our cells to stop growing and start breaking down unnecessary parts – this is the self-cleansing pathway of autophagy. Here's the critical part. If we have *diseases of excessive growth*, then we can reduce growth signaling by activating these nutrient sensors. This list of diseases includes – obesity, type 2 diabetes, Alzheimer's disease, cancer, atherosclerosis (heart attacks and strokes), polycystic ovarian syndrome, polycystic kidney disease, and fatty liver disease, among others. All these diseases are amenable to *dietary intervention, not more drugs*".[11]

Analyzing each pathway of autophagy, you probably never heard of mTOR or AMPK, but I can bet that you are very aware of the term insulin. mTOR stands for the mechanistic or mammalian target of rapamycin and its definition it's pretty complicated to understand, as it involves nutrition and medical terms which you are probably not aware of. However, a common definition would sound like this: "A protein that helps control several cell functions, including cell division and survival, and binds to rapamycin and other drugs. mTOR may be more active in some types of cancer cells than it is in normal cells. Blocking

---

11 Fung, Jason. "Autophagy – a Cure for Many Present-Day Diseases?" *Diet Doctor*, 19 Dec. 2017, www.dietdoctor.com/autophagy-cure-many-present-day-diseases.

mTOR may cause cancer cells to die. It is a type of serine/threonine protein kinase".[12]

AMPK is another difficult term to understand, as it's something similar enough to mTOR. "AMP-activated protein kinase (AMPK) is an energy sensor that regulates cellular metabolism. When activated by a deficit in nutrient status, AMPK stimulates glucose uptake and lipid oxidation to produce energy, while turning off energy-consuming processes including glucose and lipid production to restore energy balance. AMPK controls whole-body glucose homeostasis by regulating metabolism in multiple peripheral tissues, such as skeletal muscle, liver, adipose tissues, and pancreatic β cells — key tissues in the pathogenesis of type 2 diabetes. By responding to diverse hormonal signals including leptin and adiponectin, AMPK serves as an intertissue signal integrator among peripheral tissues, as well as the hypothalamus, in the control of whole-body energy balance."[13]

If there are 3 pathways for the autophagy process, there are also several types of autophagy like microautophagy, macroautophagy, and chaperone-mediated autophagy. "Macroautophagy is 'an evolutionarily conserved catabolic process involving the formation of vesicles (autophagosomes) that engulf cellular macromolecules and organelles.' This is usually the type we hear the most about. Humans are not the only species to benefit from autophagy. In fact, autophagy has been

12 "NCI Dictionary of Cancer Terms." *National Cancer Institute*, www.cancer.gov/publications/dictionaries/cancer-terms/def/mtor.

13 Long, Yun Chau, and Juleen R Zierath. "AMP-Activated Protein Kinase Signaling in Metabolic Regulation." *The Journal of Clinical Investigation*, American Society for Clinical Investigation, 3 July 2006, www.ncbi.nlm.nih.gov/pmc/articles/PMC1483147/.

observed in yeast, mold, plants, worms, flies, and mammals. Much of the research to date on autophagy has involved rats and yeast. At least 32 different autophagy-related genes (Atg) have been identified by genetic screening studies. Research continues to show that autophagic process is very important responses to starvation and stress across many species".[14]

As you probably know, insulin is a hormone responsible for allowing glucose in your blood to enter your cells and energize them to functioning properly. The more glucose you get, the more likely it is to get stored in your blood and to raise the blood sugar and insulin levels. Paradoxically speaking, higher levels of insulin will not mean a more active hormone. Only after its level *decreases* does insulin get active and starts to "work its magic," regulating the blood sugar level.

These are the pathways of autophagy, but have you ever wondered what kind of foods you need to eat in order to induce autophagy? As you can imagine, all the food you need to eat has to be low carb. You can see below a list of foods and drinks which are known to induce autophagy:

- berries and other fruits: cherries, cranberries, elderberries, blackberries, strawberries, blueberries, and raspberries
- herbs and spices: rosemary, basil, coriander, cilantro, thyme, parsley, cardamom, cumin, turmeric, cinnamon, ginger, ginseng, black pepper, and cayenne pepper
- drinks: coffee and tea. Coffee needs to be without anything, so no sugar, milk or cream. The same rule applies to tea, but it's better to

---

14 Levy, Jillian. "Benefits of Autophagy, Plus How to Induce It." *Dr. Axe*, 4 Sept. 2018, draxe.com/benefits-of-autophagy/.

be herbal, black or green tea. Try to avoid fruit tea, as it's too sweet. You can also have apple cider and distilled vinegar

- alcoholic drinks: red and white wine, gin, vermouth, and vodka.

These are just a few food and drink types you can try for inducing the autophagy process, but you may also try to some other ones which are very healthy for your body. You can find them grouped below:

- veggies (tomato, squash, spinach, peas, pickles, bell pepper, green beans, beetroot, turnip, and carrots)

- fruits (avocado, olive, coconut, watermelon, honeydew, cantaloupe)

- nuts and seeds: almonds, Brazil nuts, cashews, chestnuts, chia seeds, flax seeds, hazelnuts, Macadamia nuts, peanuts, pecans, pine nuts, pistachios, pumpkin seeds, sesame seeds, sunflower seeds, walnuts

- almond butter, peanut butter, cashew butter, Macadamia nut butter

- milk and dairy: buttermilk, blue cheese, brie cheese, cheddar cheese, Colby cheese, cottage cheese, cream cheese, feta cheese, Monterey Jack cheese, Mozzarella, Parmesan, Swiss cheese, Mascarpone, cream, heavy cream, sour cream, whole milk, skimmed milk

- fats: butter, ghee, lard, beef tallow, avocado oil, cocoa butter, coconut oil, flaxseed oil, Macadamia oil, MCT oil, olive oil, red palm oil, coconut cream, coconut milk

- drinks: almond milk, almond water, coconut water, coconut milk, kombucha;

- protein shakes with water: whey protein shake, rice protein shake, hemp protein shake, pea protein shake, micro greens blend

- alcoholic drinks: beer, champagne, rum, cognac, tequila, chocolate liquor, mint liquor

Chapter 6:

How to Start Intermittent Fasting?

You are probably not satisfied with the previous diets you had, as they were probably too radical, or they just didn't deliver the results you expected. Promising 10 or 20 pounds per week in weight loss is something very bold, which first of all, doesn't apply to all bodies. Therefore, having the right expectations is really important. Always keep in mind that most diets are to be followed on a short term basis, as they don't provide health benefits, but on the contrary, they can even do some damage to your overall health. On top of that, immediately after breaking the diet, you will start to gain weight again. So you lose weight only as long as you are on a diet.

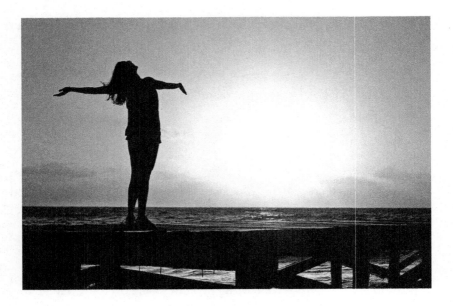

Processed food is abundant nowadays, and causes obesity on a large scale. A sedentary lifestyle combined with consuming so much processed food, and stress added, can lead to obesity. However, you don't have to be obese to start practicing intermittent fasting. One of the main principles of this way of eating is to focus on health, rather than the fat loss process itself. It's believed that a healthy body is more likely to function properly and even lose weight, so that's why IF is conducive to a healthy and sustainable weight loss. There are plenty of programs you can try when it comes to intermittent fasting, but you also need to know some important facts related to this practice:

- IF is more of a lifestyle, so it's way more than a diet
- it doesn't involve any meal requirements, as it's more about scheduling your meals, than what you eat
- don't expect miracles in terms of the weight loss process, as you will not have spectacular results. However, the fat burning process is more sustainable and a lot healthier than other diets
- it's highly recommendable to associate intermittent fasting with exercising;
- although there is no mention of any food requirements, it's highly recommendable eat healthy food, so trying a Mediterranean, keto or alkaline diet may be very good for this procedure

Such a procedure can be practiced by most people, depending on the program you choose to follow. However, some persons are not eligible for this practice:

- Pregnant women. Food deprivation is not something recommended for this category, as this is not the time to restrain themselves from food.
- Breastfeeding women. When they are breastfeeding, women really need all the possible nutrients they can get from food, so the babies get the best from breast milk.

- Women with an eating disorder like anorexia. When you are already underweight, you shouldn't be practicing intermittent fasting, as the process can lead you to even further weight loss, which may not be healthy.
- Underaged women. A growing body needs all the nutrients it can get from healthy food. Food deprivation is really not recommended in this case.

Depending on what exactly you are looking for, you can choose from any one of the intermittent fasting programs. If you prefer the daily fast, as you don't feel capable of fasting for a longer period, then perhaps the Leangains program is the right one for you. You have 8 hours to eat, and 16 hours of fasting. Daily fasts can be effective, especially if you associate it with an intense workout. Women can try cardio or endurance workouts, but swimming, jogging, Pilates and other types of physical activity are really recommended in this situation. If you feel that you can fast for more than 16 hours, then you can try the Warrior Diet, which is like an extension of the Leangains program. It limits the feeding window to just 4 hours, so you have 20 hours of the daily fast. If the previous program requires you to skip a meal, with the Warrior Diet you can only include 1 meal because you simply can't include any other main meal in just 4 hours. You can also add a snack, but still, the diet is too radical to be suitable for all women.

If you fancy fasting for a longer period, you can try the Alternate Day Fast, which includes 36 hours of fasting, or you can try the 24 hour fast. How frequent you want to have fasting days during your week is entirely up to you. For better results, you may need to add as many as possible. The Alternate Day Fast may induce autophagy, but to be sure you may need to try water fasting for 2-3 days once in a while. The second day of water fasting may be the hardest one, as you feel the most hunger. It's only up to your mind how you set it to overcome the situation and ignore the hunger. If you keep your mind occupied, you might get used to fasting, as you will not be tempted to eat and therefore, you will be able to keep on fasting. There are some side effects when it comes to fasting for a longer period, and you will experience fatigue, dizziness, and hunger. The secret to overcoming them is in your mind. If you are ambitious enough, if you are able to think of something other than the food, at some point you will get used to the fasting process, so you will no longer experience the situations mentioned above.

Intermittent fasting has plenty of benefits, but also a few side effects. You may need to try more programs to find out the one that best suits your needs. Trying a daily fasting program, associated with physical exercise and keto or Mediterranean diet can have better results in terms of fat loss, than trying a water fasting program for a long period. When you are on a water fasting program, if you do exercise, you won't have optimal performance, so your workout will not be very effective. A program which works wonders for another person, may not deliver the same results to you, or it will not have the results you expect. That's why you may need to try the several programs, before finding the one that fits your needs.

Probably the first one you will need to try is the 24 hour fast, but practiced just once a week. With intermittent fasting you will need to ease into it, so don't rush to try the hardest program, as you may not be up to it at first. After trying the 24 hour fast on a weekly basis (you can try it 3 or 4 weeks), you can switch to the Alternate Day Fast, but the mild version, as described by Dr. James B. Johnson, having just a few calories in the fasting days (or Down Days; it should be around 20% of the normal calorie consumption in the first weeks, then you can increase it to 35%). If you want to try fasting on a daily basis, you can try the Leangains program, which includes some meal scheduling for the feeding period. You will have 16 hours of daily fast, and if that's not enough, you can expand the fasting period to 20 hours per day, and transform your program into the Warrior Diet. You should try water fasting for a long period only as a last case scenario if you notice that these programs are not effective enough for you. However, you need the supervision of a physician to go on a water fasting for a longer period. Some people are able to fast for hundreds of days, consuming nothing but water and vitamins. Most doctors would not recommend water fasting for more than 72 hours, and if they consider that you need more than that, you definitely need their support and supervision in order to continue fasting for a longer period.

This is the recommended order to try the intermittent fasting programs in, but it's up to you how well you adapt to these programs. IF schedules the meals, but success also depends on what you eat, and if you work out. Combining all of these can have spectacular effects on your body, not only in terms of fat loss, but also in terms of overall health.

Chapter 7:

Focus on Healthy Food

The human body needs macronutrients, minerals, and vitamins to function properly. All of them can be found in food, but unfortunately, the food available nowadays is not very consistent in nutrients. Most of the food we eat today is processed, and the more processed food is, the more unhealthy and less consistent in nutrients. Also, processed food is rich in carbs, a macronutrient which can cause terrible effects to the human body. In fact, food has killed more people over the last few decades than drugs, alcohol, and cigarettes put together. Around 70% of the diseases known today are caused by food.

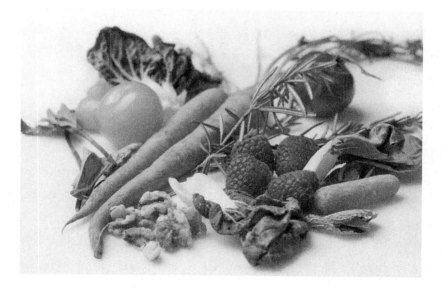

You are probably asking yourself why is this happening? The answer lies with processed foods and carbs, as they are the roots of all these problems. Carbs can be split into sugar and starch, and sugar really needs no introduction, as it's perhaps the most harmful substance ever to be consumed by humans. Without any doubt, food was a lot healthier 100 years ago, and there weren't so many cases of obesity and diabetes (both caused by an excess of carbs). The problem with sugar is that we consume it voluntarily and even feed it to our children. This kind of food causes addiction, as you will not feel satiety for a long time (in fact, you will feel hungry sooner), it won't cover the body's nutritional needs and you will crave some more carbs very soon. Those carbs contain glucose, which can be used by the body to generate energy, but this energy is produced only through physical exercise. The glucose doesn't get consumed and instead gets stored in your blood, raising your insulin and blood sugar levels. This is one step closer to diabetes, so this is how it all gets started.

Most of the food we consume today is processed and even what it claims to be natural is not organic. Before being able to process food, the most processed food you can dream of was bread, but the recipe was pretty simplistic, so different than the bread we are consuming today. Food was cooked from natural ingredients, and it had great nutritional value. Also, the lifestyle was a lot more active, as there weren't too many means of transportation back then. When we think of natural food nowadays, it's simply very difficult to find organic food, as chemicals are used to grow fruits, vegetables or crops. Fertilizers are no longer natural (with high chemical content), and animals are being fed concentrated food to grow incredibly fast. The meat we are consuming comes from these animals, and if they are fed this kind of food, this will affect us. Processing food is all about adding extra value to the product, otherwise, companies operating in this domain can't seem to find a way to increase their profits. It's fair to say that for the sake of profits, food processing companies are literally making poison to be consumed by the people. Everything which is packed and has more ingredients (many of them being chemicals you can't even pronounce) is processed food. This type of food is promoted by supermarkets and fast-food restaurants, as it fits perfectly with the current way of life. Finding healthy food is becoming a challenge nowadays, especially for the people who want to cut down on carbs. You are probably wondering what exactly you can eat in order to stay away from carbs.

Intermittent fasting is a procedure of self-discipline, in which you impose on yourself a strict set of rules and eat only within the designated feeding window. For most of the programs, there is no mention of what you can eat, however, this doesn't mean that you can stuff yourself with junk food. Healthy food can improve the results of this program, and there are a few options when it comes to healthy diets. You can consider a keto diet, a Mediterranean diet or an alkaline diet, and they all involve consuming plenty of vegetables and less meat. Most of them are LCHF (low carb high fat) diets, but the protein intake may vary from one diet to another. More details on the keto diet will be discussed in a future chapter of this book, but you can also consider utilizing a very well-balanced diet like the Mediterranean diet. This diet traces its roots from the living habits of the people living in the Mediterranean basin, so it doesn't mean just Italian cuisine. But be careful, as this diet doesn't include pizza and it doesn't focus on pasta. This kind of diet has its very own food pyramid, based on how frequent you should try that food type. If the standard food pyramid has 6 different levels like:

1) Vegetables, salad, and fruits
2) Bread, whole-grain cereals, pasta, potatoes, and rice - the food category richest in carbs
3) Milk, yogurt and cheese
4) Meat, poultry, fish, eggs, beans, and nuts

5) Oils, spread, and fats
6) Sweets, snacks, soft drinks, juices - basically food and drinks with very high levels of sugar and salt

The Mediterranean diet has it figured differently, as you can see below:

1) The base of the pyramid is represented by the physical activity, as this is a lifestyle for people living in the Mediterranean region.
2) The second level of the pyramid includes different types of food like fruits, vegetables, beans, nuts, olive oil, seeds and legumes, herbs and spices, but also grains (with a focus on whole grains). Most of the foods on this level should be consumed on a daily basis.
3) The third level of the pyramid is represented by seafood and fish, which should be consumed approximately twice a week.
4) The next level features poultry, cheese, yogurt, and eggs.
5) The last level of the pyramid is represented by meat and sweets.

The logic behind this pyramid is the same as with the standard food pyramid, the more necessary the food type is, the lower is on the pyramid. The Mediterranean diet includes a plethora of food types to choose from, all healthy, delicious and nutritious. Therefore, it's probably the most complete meal plan you can associate with intermittent fasting. You can eat fish, seafood, meat, chicken, turkey, but most of all, you will need to consume veggies, fruits, seeds, nuts, dairy products, and also olive oil. This diet focuses on healthy unsaturated fats, so it's exactly what the body needs for the IF lifestyle, as it can bring your body into ketosis (the metabolic state when ketones are multiplying to break down the fat tissue). Some of the main features of the Mediterranean diet are:

- focus on the consumption of fruits, nuts, veggies, legumes, and whole grains
- there is also a high emphasis on consuming healthy fats from canola or olive oil
- forget about the use of salt to flavor your food, as this diet encourages the use of herbs and spices
- less red meat (pork or beef) and more fish or chicken/turkey
- you can even drink red wine in moderate quantities

It doesn't sound like a diet at all, as there are so many types of food accepted. It's more of a lifestyle than a meal plan. If a standard diet is something you need to stick to for a few weeks, the Mediterranean diet is the meal plan that you have to stick to for the rest of your life. It can include all 3 meals of the day, but you can also have snacks or desserts. Sounds too good to be true? Well, this is what the Mediterranean diet is, and it can work wonders on you if you combine it with intermittent fasting and working out. But, that's not all! By now you already know the benefits of intermittent fasting. How about adding some more benefits by following this type of diet? If you want stronger bones, lower risk of frailty, lung disease or heart disease, and even to ward off depression, then you definitely need to try this diet.

Since this meal plan is very diversified, you don't have to make radical changes in your refrigerator, as you are probably already consuming some of the foods mentioned here. However, at least when it comes to veggies, legumes, and fruits, you will need to eat them fresh, so frequent shopping may be required. You need to know that the ingredients of the Mediterranean diet are structured into 11 categories, as you can see below:

1) **Vegetables** are one of the most important categories included in this meal plan and you can consume them frozen or fresh. In the frozen veggies group there can be included peas, green beans, spinach or others. In terms of fresh vegetables, you can buy tomatoes, cucumbers, peppers, onions, okra, green beans, zucchini, garlic, peas, cauliflower, mushrooms, broccoli, potatoes, peas, carrots, celery leaves, cabbage, spinach, beets, or romaine lettuce.

2) The **fruits** you need to include in your shopping list are peaches, pears, figs, apricots, apples, oranges, tangerines, lemons, cherries, and watermelon.

3) You can't have a Mediterranean diet without some high-fat **dairy** products. Milk (whether is whole or semi-skimmed) is no longer considered a good option, as it also has a higher concentration of carbs. You can buy instead sheep's milk yogurt, Greek yogurt, feta cheese, ricotta (or other types of fresh cheese), mozzarella, graviera, and mizithra.

4) This diet doesn't focus too much on **meat or poultry,** but you can still eat them twice a week. Your shopping list will need to include chicken (whether you prefer it whole, breasts or thighs), pork, ground beef, and veal. This is where you can get most of your proteins from, but still, you need to keep the protein intake at a low level.

5) Can you imagine a Mediterranean diet without **fish or seafood**? Because this food type is a must in this meal plan, although you only have it twice a week. So, you will need to buy salmon, tuna, cod, sardines, anchovies, shrimp, octopus or calamari. You can eat some of them fresh or canned.

6) Although you don't have to abuse them, your shopping list should definitely include **bread or pasta**. If they are made from whole

grains even better, as they are the right choice in this case. Try to avoid the unnecessary consumption of pastry, like having bagels, pretzels or croissants with your coffee. You can eat and buy instead whole grains bread, paximadi (barley rusks), breadsticks (also made from whole grains), pita bread, phyllo, pasta, rice, egg pasta, bulgur, and couscous.

7) Your shopping list must include **healthy fats and nuts**. Olive oil should be consumed on a daily basis, so you need to have it in your household. Also, in terms of nuts, it's recommended that you buy tahini, almonds, walnuts, pine nuts, pistachios, and sesame seeds.

8) **Beans** are an important part of this diet, so you definitely need to buy lentils, white beans chickpeas, and fava.

9) **Pantry items** are the miscellaneous part of this meal plan. In this group, you can include olives, canned tomatoes, tomato paste, sun-dried tomatoes, capers, herbal tea, honey, balsamic or red wine vinegar and wine (preferably red).

10) As mentioned above, **herbs and spices** are used for flavoring your food. As this diet involves a lot of home cooking, having plenty of spices and herbs can make a difference. That's why your shopping list must include herbs and spices like oregano, mint, dill, parsley, cumin, basil, sea salt, black pepper, cinnamon, sea salt and all kind of spices.

11) You definitely need to buy some greens, like chicory, dandelion, beet greens and amaranth and include them in your meal plan.

Chapter 8:

Calories

Any type of processed food is literally a calorie bomb, as the food is rich in calories, but it's very poor in terms of nutrients. Eating more calorie-dense foods will not keep the hunger away for a longer time, in fact, you will feel the hunger again faster than you think. When studying the label of any processed product, we can see the nutritional value table.

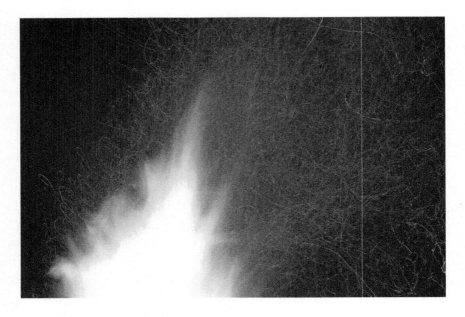

You will quickly notice that the food you are consuming is extremely rich in calories, but you will also notice really low values for proteins and sometimes even fats. Eating plenty of calories will not guarantee you extra energy, but burning them will. So why eat plenty of unnecessary calories per day, when you know that they are not going to be burned in full? You are probably wondering what is the normal calorie intake for the average woman. The answer depends on the muscle mass, height, and other factors. "An average woman needs to eat about 2000 calories per day to maintain, and 1500 calories to lose one pound of weight per week. An average man needs 2500 calories to maintain, and 2000 to lose one pound of weight per week. However, this depends on numerous factors. These include age, height, current weight, activity levels, metabolic health, and several others."[15]

Calories are units that measure energy and can be found in most food and drinks. People nowadays don't pay too much attention to how many calories they are consuming. Not only is processed food way too high in calories, but people may also snack often and drink soft drinks or juices, products which are also rich in calories. The lack of physical activity leaves too many calories unburned, and this is how the fat cells are accumulating.

Obesity is a major problem over the past few years, and unfortunately, it looks like it will continue to remain an even more serious problem in the years to come. The major problem with the food today is its quality, it is very calorie dense, not nutrient dense. It will not maintain the satiety level for a longer period, and it will make your body crave food again in short order. People often snack during such moments, and probably the most dangerous type of snack is a bag of chips. The calorie level skyrockets and more and more people have problems controlling their weight. The energy from the calories gets stored in

---

15 Gunnars, Kris. "How Many Calories Should You Eat Per Day to Lose Weight?" *Healthline*, Healthline Media, 6 July 2018, www.healthline.com/nutrition/how-many-calories-per-day#section1.

your blood (in the form of blood sugar) or in the fat tissue, where you need special help from ketones to release the energy stored in there.

If you were used to eating plenty of calories per day, then you definitely need to lower the amount to approximately 2000 calories per day, or 1500 if you are planning to lose weight. Keeping the calorie intake at this level will either maintain your weight, or you can start to lose weight. Trying intermittent fasting doesn't mean that you need to eat more calories in the feeding period in order to compensate for the calorie intake for the lack of it in the fasting period. The eating window will need to be as on a normal day, the standard calorie intake, in order to make the IF program more efficient. Below you can find some of the best tips to control your calorie intake:

- focus on natural food, not processed. Following a special diet low in carbs can be the right thing, so an alkaline, Mediterranean or keto diet might be exactly what you need to keep the control of calories
- keep track of how many calories you are consuming. Although natural food is not packed as processed food is, you still need to browse for information over the internet to find out how many calories a steak or a salad may have
- rule out junk food. This type of food is the most calorie-dense food out there, and in terms of nutrients is very poor
- if you feel the need to snack, always use fruits, veggies, nuts, or smoothies. Forget about chips and other types of processed snacks
- make sure you avoid soft drinks or juices with high sugar levels. They are also very high in calories

It's hard to resist the temptation of consuming processed food since it's so popular and readily available. Completely eliminating pizza, burgers, donuts, chips, and soft drinks can be something very hard to do, as most of us really love all these kinds of foods, and we are addicted to them. Small things can make a difference, like not using sugar, milk or cream with your coffee, or eating natural meat, instead of processed ones (like sausages or meatballs). As a word of advice, don't even bother with reading the label of processed food. It will literally scare you because of the very high calorie level. Instead, shop around for fruits, veggies, and meat (although you don't have to eat too much of it). In many cases, when you have a steak, you shouldn't have French fries (or any type of cooked potatoes) or rice as a side dish, since these foods are rich in carbs and also high in calories. Instead have some grilled veggies (like peas, broccoli, carrots, and so on), and this should significantly lower the calorie intake of that meal. By the way, meat shouldn't be consumed on a daily basis, and even when you consume it, try to avoid frying it in oil (vegetable or sunflower oil). A keto diet should help you a lot with the calorie intake, but more details regarding this very popular diet can be found in the next chapter.

Chapter 9:

Keto Diet

If you want to better understand why you need to follow a ketogenic diet, you need to first understand terms like ketosis and ketones. "Ketosis is a metabolic state in which your body uses fat and ketones rather than glucose (sugar) as its main fuel source. Glucose is stored in your liver and released as needed for energy.

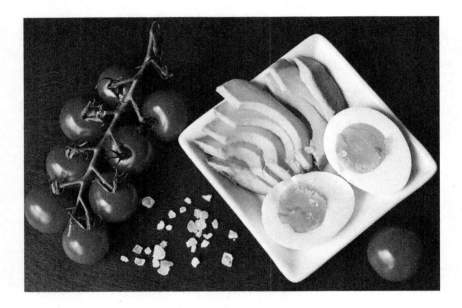

However, after carb intake has been extremely low for one to two days, these glucose stores become depleted. Your liver can make some glucose from amino acids in the protein you eat via a process known as gluconeogenesis, but not nearly enough to meet the needs of your brain, which requires a constant fuel supply. Fortunately, ketosis can provide you with an alternative source of energy".[16]

However, some specialists would disagree. They claim that ketosis is just the metabolic state with appropriate levels of insulin and ketones and the keto-adapted state is what makes the body run on fats.

Speaking of ketones, there are a few things you need to understand. "In ketosis, your body produces ketones at an accelerated rate. Ketones, or ketone bodies, are made by your liver from fat that you eat and your own body fat. The three ketone bodies are beta-hydroxybutyrate (BHB), acetoacetate, and acetone (although acetone is technically a breakdown product of acetoacetate). Even when on a higher-carb diet, your liver actually produces ketones on a regular basis – mainly overnight while you sleep – but usually only in tiny amounts. However, when glucose and insulin levels decrease on a carb-restricted diet, the liver ramps up its production of ketones in order to provide energy for your brain. Once the level of ketones in your blood reaches a certain threshold, you are considered to be in nutritional ketosis. According to leading ketogenic diet researchers Dr. Steve Phinney and Dr. Jeff Volek, the threshold for nutritional ketosis is a minimum of 0.5 mmol/L of BHB (the ketone body measured in the blood)".[17]

---

16 Spritzler, Franziska, and Andreas Eenfeldt. "What Is Ketosis? Is It Safe? – Diet Doctor." *Diet Doctor*, 22 Mar. 2019, www.dietdoctor.com/low-carb/ketosis.

17 Spritzler, Franziska, and Andreas Eenfeldt. "What Is Ketosis? Is It Safe? – Diet Doctor." *Diet Doctor*, 22 Mar. 2019, www.dietdoctor.com/low-carb/ketosis.

Now that we have this covered, the keto diet is one of the low carb high fat (LCHF) meal plans, and it is definitely one of the most popular diets nowadays. If done correctly, this dietary plan should provide you amazing results in terms of health management and weight loss. Just like intermittent fasting, the keto diet puts health first, as it's important for the body to achieve the right health status. You are probably wondering, what's the secret of this amazing diet? What exactly made it so famous? I will try to explain to you in this chapter, so you can easily understand its popularity.

The ketogenic diet is capable of reprogramming your body to run on fats instead of glucose, therefore it will burn body fat for energy, instead of glucose from carbs. The default fuel type of the body is glucose, especially with the food we eat today. You can find plenty of glucose in bread, pasta, potatoes, rice and all kinds of processed food. Unfortunately, almost everything we eat has a high or very high carb concentration. But, it's not just what we eat, it's also what we drink. Just think of all the juices and soft drinks with high sugar levels. So, glucose can come from carbs (when we consume too many of them), but it can also come from proteins. In other words, most of the food we eat today is very high in glucose. Energy comes from burning glucose, not from consuming it, so you will need to engage in physical activities in order to burn glucose, otherwise, it will get stored in your blood. This can lead to higher blood sugar, and this is where it all gets started when it comes to diabetes. Therefore, consuming high amounts of glucose is definitely not healthy for your body, so you need to find a way to replace it with a different energy source.

The ketogenic diet can provide you the alternative, as it's capable of replacing the carbs from your dietary plan with healthy fats. The ironic

174

part is that you will lose weight. That's right! You will eat fat and lose weight! That's how the ketogenic diet works.

If you are wondering how this is possible, let me break it down for you. In the beginning of the chapter, there were some mentions about ketosis, the keto-adapted state and of course, ketones. Let's say that you radically change your diet, and you mostly eat fats. Since your body is so used to running on glucose, it will quickly notice that there is no more glucose to burn, since it's already stored in your blood, and that's not available to be consumed (insulin will take care of the glucose stored in your blood). Applying stress like controlled hunger (through intermittent fasting), or consuming dietary fat (using a keto diet), will activate the metabolic state of ketosis. The insulin level is decreasing until it eventually gets activated, while the ketone bodies are multiplying.

Now that you are consuming high levels of fat, your body will need to adapt to find a way to turn all this fat into energy. This is what the ketones are for. They are the only ones capable of breaking down fats and releasing the energy stored in there. Fats are easier to burn using the action of ketones than it was with glucose through physical activity. Switching the fuel type from carbs to fats is not easy. Although the modern Western diet is very poor in terms of nutrients (just rich in carbs) and you will not feel satiety for a long time, your body will crave more carbs once you feel hungry. At this point, it's addicted to carbs, so switching the fuel type to fats may not be something that it enjoys at first. There are plenty of reasons why you should cut down on carbs and replace them with fats. Once your body realizes that there is no more glucose to use, it will start burning fat for energy using ketones. If you don't eat anything, the ketones will act on your fat tissue, but if you eat keto food, it will burn through the dietary fat. Unlike glucose, which is no longer available once it gets stored in your blood, fats can be consumed and burned if they are already stored in your fat tissue, or if you just ate them. Once you have your body running on fats, keep feeding it mostly fats, and it will continue to run on this "fuel type." Just think of fats as the "biofuel" your body can use, as it will enhance your longevity, but it will also improve the function of your "engine" (which is the heart).

Speaking of benefits, you definitely need to check them below, just to have extra motivation to make this radical change to your diet.

The Benefits of the Ketogenic Diet

So far, we established the effects the keto diet has on your weight. You will start to lose weight once you switch to this diet. You can even try working out, to lose more weight and to accelerate the fat-burning process, but you also need to have the right expectations, as the keto diet is not a meal plan selling you false promises. Don't expect to lose 10 or 20 pounds per week. However, you will be able to notice some pleasant results once you climb on your scale.

It lowers the risk of prediabetes and diabetes

When dealing with such diseases and medical conditions, it's highly important to understand terms like insulin and high blood sugar. The modern Western diet "helps" you consume too much glucose, which will not get used (at least not all of it) and it will get stored in your blood. This is raising your blood sugar level until is too high above normal, which is a condition called high blood sugar, or in medical terms hyperglycemia. However, the body has the means to fight back (if you let it), so the pancreas can release insulin, which is a peptide hormone capable of lowering down the blood sugar level. Consuming too much glucose will also raise the insulin level, and the body becomes insulin resistant. In this phase, the insulin is not capable of fighting against the sugar (glucose) stored in your blood. Something has to change in order to reactivate the insulin.

Stopping the intake of glucose through intermittent fasting, or in this case, through the keto diet is exactly the kind of help insulin needs in order to get activated again, and to regulate the blood sugar level. In other words, glucose consumption is the cause, and the keto diet simply eliminates the cause and encourages the body to fight back using insulin. Although carbs may not be completely removed from your body, the glucose intake will be too low, and therefore it will be consumed immediately (and entirely), so you don't have to worry about getting more of it to your blood. The percentage of a keto meal plan should be at 75% fats, just 5 -10 % carbs, and the rest should be proteins. Obesity goes hand in hand with different medical conditions like diabetes, heart diseases, and many others. When you see the ads on social media, promoting all kind of diets promising you to lose 10-20 pounds per week guaranteed, what proof you have to support that?

As it turns out, all the benefits of the keto diet are backed up by science, so there were actual studies showing what results you can expect. There was a study conducted which concluded that people on a keto diet managed to lose 24.4 pounds, compared to 15.2 pounds lost by the people from the non-keto group (don't expect these results in a week, as the study was conducted for a period longer than a month). On top of that, 95% of the people on this diet were able to cut down on most of their diabetes medication, compared to just 62% of the people from the non-keto group. Another study also discovered a very interesting fact about the keto diet and diabetes: 7 people out of 21 renounced all diabetes medication after trying this diet.

The benefits of the keto diet don't apply just to weight loss and diabetes. There are plenty of other diseases or medical conditions which can be impacted by this dietary plan, as you can see below:

- Heart disease. Less body fat means a lower cholesterol level, but it can also lead to lower blood pressure and blood sugar. Therefore, the keto diet has a positive impact on blood circulation, and it can play an important role when it comes to preventing heart disease.

- Cancer. Remember, the keto diet can lead to autophagy and as mentioned in the prior chapter about this process, autophagy can prevent and even reverse cancer in an incipient phase. The ketogenic diet is capable of slowing down tumor growth, but also other types of cancer, assuming that they are in an incipient phase. There are plenty of cases when cancer is caused by the food we eat. Consuming healthy food is something highly recommended, and can help you prevent a terrible disease like cancer.

- Parkinson's and Alzheimer's diseases. Although it may sound a bit much, the keto diet is known to improve cognitive and mental function, therefore it can slow the progression of or even prevent neurodegenerative diseases like Alzheimer's and Parkinson's.

- Epilepsy. Several studies have shown the positive impact the keto diet has in reducing seizures for epileptic children, and also for adults.

- Polycystic ovarian syndrome can be caused by high insulin levels. Since the keto diet restricts carb consumption, this means that you will significantly lower the level of glucose. Lowering the glucose level will eventually lower the insulin level as well, and there will be a lower risk of polycystic ovarian syndrome.

- Brain injuries. Although the study was conducted on animals, the result is valid for humans too. There was a research that proved that the keto diet is able to decrease the effects of concussions and it can contribute to lower the recovery time after a brain injury.

- Acne. This condition may be caused by the excess of glucose in your blood. Since the keto diet is known for reducing the blood sugar and insulin levels, it can help with improving acne, and also other skin conditions. You can also induce autophagy by sticking to this diet, and this process has very impressive results on your skin, as it recycles and replaces the parts of the old cells, including at a skin level.

These benefits should determine everyone to radically change their meal plan and switch to the keto diet. However, you will probably need to make some serious changes in your refrigerator and your spices cabinet as your shopping list must include: almond butter, almond milk, almond butter, beef sticks (you must check the label for the carbs count), beef jerky, blackberries, cocoa nibs, cheese wedges, cheese slices, cheese chips, Brazil nuts, coconut oil, deli meat, dark chocolate, Greek yogurt, flaxseed crackers, cottage cheese, kale chips, Macadamia nuts, sugar-free Jell-O, olives, meat bars, Macadamia nut butter, peanut butter, pickles, pecans, pepperoni slices, protein bars (keep an eye on the carbs level), pork rinds, pumpkin seeds, seaweed snacks, sardines, smoked oysters, sunflower seeds, eggs, string cheese, walnuts, cauliflower, broccoli, avocado, mushrooms, toasted coconut flakes, string cheese, guacamole (pay extra attention to the carb levels), peppers and many other fruits or vegetables.

The fun part with the keto diet is that you can have all of the main meals, plus desserts and snacks. There are plenty of books providing plenty of keto recipes. You can follow them and prepare really delicious and nutritious food. Usually, people associate snacks with a very unhealthy habit of eating chips, sweets and drinking juices or soft drinks with very high sugar intake. The big problem with the modern-day diet is that the food is only calorie dense, not nutrient dense. It gives you the false impression of satiety, but that will not last for long. Carbs can cause addiction, and you will not feel satisfied, so you will need to eat more carbs. Even though it may be a challenge, there are snacks and desserts which are keto, so they are high in fats and low in carbs. Snacks and desserts can perpetuate the metabolic state of ketosis, as you will consume more fats. The keto diet can be a very important part of the "health triad", 3 elements that can help you become more healthy and lose more weight. The 3 elements of this health triad are intermittent fasting, the keto diet and physical exercise. All these combined can help your body enter ketosis, can help with the keto-adaptation process and eventually induce autophagy. Whether you want to combine this meal plan with IF and exercising, or you would like to stick just to the keto diet, you will experience plenty of benefits by trying this dietary plan.

Chapter 10:

Muscle Gain

Intermittent fasting means food deprivation, and you need a daily intake to maintain your muscle mass. People mostly think that this procedure will cause muscle loss, not just fat burning. Well, they couldn't be more wrong! You are probably asking yourself, how is this even possible? Even though you are not eating the daily recommended intake of protein required to preserve your muscles, you will still not lose any muscle mass. Let me explain why.

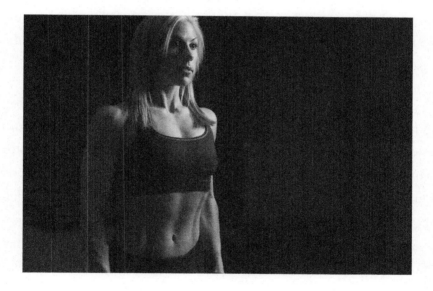

When people tell you that they want to lose weight, they want to lose *fat*. Most of the studies on this indicate that intermittent fasting programs are conducive for losing weight. However, the question you need to ask yourself is what kind of weight are you willing to lose? Losing muscle is not something that you can benefit from in most cases, so you are definitely wanting just to lose fat.

Physical exercise is highly important, as it can make the difference between losing muscles and fat, or losing just fat. Without exercise, you can lose the whole package through intermittent fasting, so you can experience both lean mass and fat mass loss. The lean mass includes the muscles as well. Working out can turn fats into muscles, so you can at least preserve or even expand your muscle mass through physical exercise. If you pair it with IF, then most likely your body will burn fat on a massive scale and will preserve your muscles. You will probably need to try high-intensity workouts in order to avoid muscle loss, but you will also need to remember that the growth hormone levels get very high through intermittent fasting. For example, after 48 hours of continuous fasting, the growth hormone level is 5 times higher than the one during the feeding window. This explains how your body will not lose weight if you work out intensely during the fasting period.

If you think about it, the prehistoric humans fasted a lot because they didn't have 3 main meals during the day, and it took a long time from one meal to another. They needed to hunt, fish or eat all sorts of foods, which were scarce and required some skills to acquire. The prehistoric human was a lot stronger than the modern-day human, even though they had to fast for longer periods. They had proper nutrient-dense food and had a very active lifestyle (which involved plenty of running, climbing trees or swimming). This is how intermittent fasting with exercise can be a very good combination to become stronger. Although there are better methods to gain weight, IF can prove to be a very effective way to pile on some muscle.

Several studies were conducted to find out how the human body reacts to food deprivation, so now we have some results of how the body reacts in a fasted state.

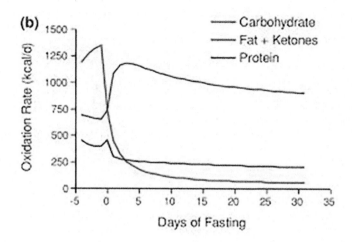

(b) Oxidation Rate (kcal/d) vs Days of Fasting

Legend: Carbohydrate, Fat + Ketones, Protein

The graph above is taken from the "Comparative Physiology of Fasting, Starvation and Food Limitation" by Dr. Kevin Hall. It clearly shows where the energy is coming from in different moments of intermittent fasting. You can also notice that the body is using a mix of energy sources, mainly from carbs at the beginning, and then it uses the energy from fat and ketones. "Within the first day or so of fasting, the body initially continues burning stored carbs for energy. Though, you'll notice that shortly after the body burns through those stored carbs it beings burning fat. This fat burning state is what drives diets like the Ketogenic diet. Meaning that in the absence of carbs your body has turned to a sort of 'backup generator' for energy, which is stored fat. So what about the protein (AKA muscle)? Well, while there is a low baseline of protein consumption there is no big spike in your body feasting on your muscle. In fact, this lowered baseline is an indicator of your body conserving muscle. Meaning that being in a fasted state doesn't automatically make your muscle wither away". [18]

18 George, Lesley. "Intermittent Fasting And Muscle Gain: Go To Guide To Fasting Like A Pro • Shapezine - Digital Health & Fitness

Just like we mentioned above, gaining muscle mass through intermittent fasting may not be the best method, but it's still possible. You will need to set the right conditions and environment for your muscles to grow. This is why you need to make sure you have 3 factors in place: sufficient resources, a positive nitrogen balance and the third one is to apply enough stress to the muscle mass in order to achieve hypertrophy.

The necessary resource for your body in terms of muscle growth is protein. Under normal circumstances, you will need to consume more proteins to gain more muscles. That's why bodybuilders stuff themselves with protein shakes or bars. However, during fasting, the situation is totally different. So it can get you confused and it will definitely make you wonder: "How can I be providing my body with enough food to grow muscle when I'm fasting? Well, providing your body with resources is more about the quantity of food rather than the timing. Meaning that you could fast for 8 hours in the morning then consume your caloric goal of 2,000 calories in the evening. Still maintaining that fasted state while also consuming enough calories to properly recover."[19]

Tracking Blog." *Shapezine - Digital Health & Fitness Tracking Blog*, 10 July 2018, shapescale.com/blog/health/intermittent-fasting-muscle-gain/.

19 George, Lesley. "Intermittent Fasting And Muscle Gain: Go To Guide To Fasting Like A Pro • Shapezine - Digital Health & Fitness Tracking Blog." *Shapezine - Digital Health & Fitness Tracking Blog*, 10

When it comes to the positive nitrogen balance, it's all about eating more proteins than it is eliminating. So you need to make sure that you assimilate proteins and you are not eliminating them through urine. This will eventually lead to muscle growth, so digesting proteins is what you need.

"Therefore, if we want to make sure we're in a positive nitrogen balance, we must simply consume enough protein. What this means for someone who is fasting is: consume enough calories during our 'feeding window' and pack in the protein. It's essentially the same as above. Just because you have a smaller window to consume protein doesn't mean you can't get enough. This way of eating simply concentrates your protein intake to a certain period. Instead of throughout the day."[20]

Have you ever wondered what the best way to gain muscles through training is? The answer is simple. You will need to use heavier weights, as applying more stress to the muscles will favor their growth. Make sure you add as much weight as you can lift, so try not to over-exaggerate, as you definitely want to avoid accidents or even hernias. Some specialists would agree that trying HIIT is the best way to grow your muscles through training. This involves having just a few repeats with very heavy weights for about 20 seconds, then have 10 seconds

July 2018, shapescale.com/blog/health/intermittent-fasting-muscle-gain/.

20 George, Lesley. "Intermittent Fasting And Muscle Gain: Go To Guide To Fasting Like A Pro • Shapezine - Digital Health & Fitness Tracking Blog." *Shapezine - Digital Health & Fitness Tracking Blog*, 10 July 2018, shapescale.com/blog/health/intermittent-fasting-muscle-gain/.

break, then repeating the whole process again 8 times. So in 4 minutes, you can work a group of muscles very intensely. Others recommend progressive overload, which "means increasing the stress placed on the muscle through added weight. There are a number of ways that you can achieve progressive overload. However, the main two are: adding weight to the bar without sacrificing sets and reps or adding reps without sacrificing weight or sets. These are both great recipes to achieve efficient muscle growth. If you are achieving the above two factors of enough calories and protein, then there is no reason to have issues in progressing in your workouts. Even if you are actively practicing fasting."[21]

All of the conditions above set the right environment for your muscles to grow during intermittent fasting, whilst you are in the fasted state. Therefore, you will need to make sure that you will only get rid of the excess fat, not the muscle mass. You definitely need to work out very intensely, so if you want to gain muscles don't be afraid to deal with heavier weights. Having too many repetitions with lighter weights will not do you any good in terms of muscle growth. You probably don't want to develop the body of a weightlifter, but you will still need to use heavier weights for better results in terms of muscle gain.

The next thing you will need to make sure you master is the energy dosage and a very important tip is to master the caloric cycling process, which basically means setting up the quantity and timing of the eating

---

21 George, Lesley. "Intermittent Fasting And Muscle Gain: Go To Guide To Fasting Like A Pro • Shapezine - Digital Health & Fitness Tracking Blog." *Shapezine - Digital Health & Fitness Tracking Blog,* 10 July 2018, shapescale.com/blog/health/intermittent-fasting-muscle-gain/.

periods. The basic idea is to consume more calories when you train (after your exercise) and fewer calories when you don't. The best time to work out is during the fasted state, so you definitely need to avoid any kind of nutrient intake before your workout. "The key idea here being, adjust your calorie intake to help your body recover after hard workouts and don't be afraid pack in the protein. On days that you don't train you can back off on the calories. Especially, the carbs. How this translates to being incorporated into a fasting-centered diet is by simply making sure you are fitting the appropriate calories in your feeding window. Pretty simple."[22]

It's up to you to decide which intermittent fasting program works best for you in terms of muscle growth if you associate it with physical exercise. Probably the best programs are the daily fasting ones since they can provide you will all key requirements for your muscles to grow through IF. That's why the Leangains program and the Warrior Diet may be the right ones for you. Bodybuilders are huge fans of the Leangains program (also known as the 16/8 hour fast). It basically splits the day into an 8-hour feeding window and a 16-hour fasting period. This program may be the perfect example of caloric cycling, as it very clearly sets your feeding period and fasting period, but you can also plan to eat the most consistent meal of the day after your workout. If you want to burn fat and gain muscles at the same time, you can adapt your very own Leangains method:

---

22 George, Lesley. "Intermittent Fasting And Muscle Gain: Go To Guide To Fasting Like A Pro • Shapezine - Digital Health & Fitness Tracking Blog." *Shapezine - Digital Health & Fitness Tracking Blog*, 10 July 2018, shapescale.com/blog/health/intermittent-fasting-muscle-gain/.

- 8:00 - 9:15 am it can be workout time. You can train at your local gym, but don't be afraid to "play" with heavier weights.
- 10 am - the most consistent meal of the day. Forget about the typical breakfast, as you shouldn't eat cereals for breakfast. A protein boost is what you need, so a very consistent omelet with bacon and cheese seems to be the right choice.
- 2 pm - it's time for lunch. Grilled meat like chicken or pork, served with vegetables on the side can be the right choice. Don't forget about salad as an option.
- 6 pm - a light dinner. Take it easy with the calorie intake for this meal. When it comes to the meals of the day, make sure they are low on carbs, and higher on proteins and fats.

Your body should still run on fats, that's why the carb level should be at a minimum level. However, you will need to make sure that your protein intake gets assimilated by your body, and your muscles will begin to grow. Repeating the schedule above, working hard at the gym and also having the proper protein intake should definitely lead to muscle gain. To maximize your protein intake, you can also have a protein shake or bar between the meals. This is how you can make sure your muscles will grow through intermittent fasting.

Strangely enough, studies have shown that the growth hormone reaches unbelievably high levels if you fast for at least 48 hours. At that point, it's 5 times higher than it was in the feeding period. That sounds too good to be true, but most humans can't benefit from this situation, as they don't have the necessary resources at that point to engage in very intense training. If the growth hormone has very high levels, it may still not be enough to grow your muscles, as you will need intense training to take advantage of the high values of this growth hormone.

Chapter 11:

Common Mistakes

Intermittent fasting is starting to become a very popular practice, however, it's important that it be understood and applied properly in order to take advantage of all its benefits, whether we're talking about weight loss, better digestion, fewer cravings, or lower inflammation. Truth be told, you should set your fasting window for as long as *you* feel comfortable with. Using a daily fasting program might be the easiest program to stick to, as you have just 16 hours of fasting period per day, which sounds totally doable.

Other programs involve increasing the fasting window to 20, 24 or 36 hours. Only the first one can involve daily fasting, as the other ones may involve fasting for once or twice a week if you feel up to simply quitting food for a longer period of time. It's true that the Alternate Day Fast (with a fasting window of 36 hours) may allow you to consume a minimum amount of calories in the fasting period (limited to just 500 calories in that day). Other people may want to consider the "purest" IF program, which is water fasting, but only a few people are capable of sticking to this one.

Whether you prefer daily fasting or longer term fasting, should be up to you. You may need to try a few intermittent fasting programs to find out which program best suits your needs. Also, you need to set the right expectations, as this program simply can't make false promises, so you can't expect to lose 10 or 20 pounds per week. It may not be the quickest weight loss program, but you can easily consider it one of the healthiest.

It's said that humans best learn from mistakes, so you can find below a list of the most common mistakes when it comes to IF:

1) Quitting too soon. Let's face it! Intermittent fasting is simply not easy, mostly because your body will need to run on just a few calories, or without any food at all for a longer-than-usual period. It's more about self-discipline, as you need to train your body and mind to overcome the stress of food deprivation, even if you feel hungry. Once you practice this for more than a week (you can try daily fasting, not necessarily water fasting for more than a week), you will get used to it, and you will not feel as hungry and irritated anymore. If you are not reaching this phase, you probably chose the wrong IF program, and you may need to try a different one. Still, don't get discouraged, as there are high chances that one of the intermittent fasting programs might suit your needs.

2) Over-eating at meal time. This procedure will definitely make you experience hunger, but this doesn't mean that you need to stuff yourself with too much food, just because you are very hungry. Try

not to compensate for the time you are not consuming calories, as you will rule out most of the benefits of intermittent fasting, especially the one related to weight loss. Dr. Brigitte Zeitlin is one of the specialists in this field of expertise, and she believes in the healthy principle of "fewer calories in than calories out." In other words, you will need to lower your calorie intake, as if you consume the same amount of calories or even more, you will definitely not lose weight at all. This procedure should lower the amount of food you consume during the day, and this means fewer calories. "Instead of piling food onto your plate when it's finally time to eat, portion out your meals so you know exactly what you're taking in and avoid that whole 'eyes bigger than your stomach' situation. If you need a little help understanding how many calories to strive for—and what macronutrients those calories should consist of—Zeitlin suggests keeping a food journal or using an app like MyFitnessPal or Fitbit to get a clear picture of how your current food intake matches up to your goals and what nutrients you may need more or less of. And when you do sit down for your meals, take your time eating so your hunger cues have ample time to kick in and let you know if you truly need more."[23]

3) Eating insufficient amounts of food. The body still needs macronutrients, minerals, and vitamins from food in order to function properly. Intermittent fasting means food deprivation, but you don't need to overdo it. You still need to eat properly, even though you are trying any of the IF programs. This procedure is simply not for everyone, and most specialists don't recommend

---

23 Lefave, Samantha. "8 Major Mistakes People Make When Intermittent Fasting." *What's Good by V*, 31 Jan. 2019, whatsgood.vitaminshoppe.com/intermittent-fasting-mistakes/.

fasting for more than 72 hours. If someone is determined to fast for a longer period, this should only be done with the strict supervision of a physician. People should not try to radicalize this program, so they shouldn't eat too little. "'Some people don't want to undo what they've just done while fasting for hours or they have the mentality that if they eat too much the next fasting period will be harder," says Zeitlin. But consistently eating far below your calorie needs is a mistake, and kicks your body into 'starvation mode,' slowing your metabolism and making it that much harder to shed fat. Even if you're restricting when you eat your food, 'your body still needs an ample amount of food so your organs can function, and you can think straight and be the fantastic human that you are,' she says."[24] Not eating enough calories will cause you to feel irritable, weak and unable to focus.

4) Not consuming the right food. It goes without saying that some types of food should definitely be avoided. I'm referring of course to processed and junk food. Any type of packed food, with too many ingredients (some of them are impossible to pronounce) should be avoided, as they are incredibly high in carbs. However, food types like bread, pastry, pasta, potatoes, and rice should be consumed only moderately, as they also have high carb levels. Unfortunately, processed food is calorie dense and definitely not nutrient dense. This means they have too many calories compared to their nutritional value. These kinds of food will not make you feel satiety for a long time. In plenty of cases, you will feel the urge to snack soon after your last meal, and then react by consuming a

---

24 Lefave, Samantha. "8 Major Mistakes People Make When Intermittent Fasting." *What's Good by V*, 31 Jan. 2019, whatsgood.vitaminshoppe.com/intermittent-fasting-mistakes/.

bag of chips or eating some kind of sweets. Having a soft drink or a very sweet juice is probably the worst drink you can have with these snacks. It's a vicious circle because it encourages you to consume more carbs, more processed food and drinks, which will eventually affect your health. "Focus on eating a healthy balance of all the macronutrients (healthy fats, lean protein, and carbs) and fiber (which will help with satiety, gas, and bloating) your body needs to function well. Zeitlin suggests loading half your plate with veggies, a quarter with lean protein (think fish, chicken, and turkey), and a quarter with healthy starches like brown rice, quinoa, and sweet potato. If you're going to end up eating slightly fewer calories than usual, you need those calories to be as nutritious and body-serving as possible. Just because you're eating fewer calories doesn't mean those calories can come from sub-par sources."[25]

5) Not drinking enough fluids. Hydration is very important during intermittent fasting, and many beginners are thinking that they simply can't consume anything during fasting hours. Well, that's wrong! You don't have to fast strictly, leaving out water as well. In fact, there's nothing wrong with consuming water, coffee or tea during this period. However, there is a rule. Don't use any sugar, or any milk, cream or butter. In other words, don't add anything to your tea or coffee. Hydrating yourself can be a very useful tool when it comes to extending your feeling of satiety. Therefore, drinking water can help you get rid of the hunger feeling.

6) Going for the hardest program. Many people feel like they want to challenge themselves when taking on an intermittent fasting

---

25 Lefave, Samantha. "8 Major Mistakes People Make When Intermittent Fasting." *What's Good by V*, 31 Jan. 2019, whatsgood.vitaminshoppe.com/intermittent-fasting-mistakes/.

program, so they're fasting for several days during the week (I'm not referring to daily fasting, it's about fasting for at least 24 hours). The Eat-Stop-Eat program involves fasting for 24 hours twice a week, so it's fair to also call it the 5:2 program. Turning this program into 4:3, may not be something recommendable, in fact, it can even be dangerous. "'You're not supposed to starve yourself,' says Zeitlin. 'Our bodies require fuel to think straight, work well, converse normally, and move around—and that fuel comes from calories,' she says. Restricting your food intake too much takes a toll on your everyday life—and that's not what fasting is all about."[26]

7) Forcing the intermittent fasting programs. You need to understand right from the beginning that this procedure may not be the best when it comes to longevity, weight loss or metabolic health. It's a very sustainable method, but it doesn't work for everyone. Setting the right expectations is very important, as you know exactly what can be achieved through IF. That's why if you are trying an intermittent fasting program and you feel it's not delivering the results you expect, you need to stop trying this program and try another one. Starving yourself on a regular basis may not be the best way to get the benefits of this lifestyle. If you think of the prehistoric humans, they didn't have food on a regular basis, so they fasted involuntarily. For example, intermittent fasting may not be for people with strong appetites because they are not used to restraining themselves from food for a longer period of time.

---

26 Lefave, Samantha. "8 Major Mistakes People Make When Intermittent Fasting." *What's Good by V*, 31 Jan. 2019, whatsgood.vitaminshoppe.com/intermittent-fasting-mistakes/.

8) Not switching to an active lifestyle. Plenty of diets can promise you will lose many pounds, as the food type they are promoting just burns fat without any effort. This isn't quite true. You may be able to eat food which is rich in fats, but without physical activity, it's all in vain. This is the right type of stress that can make your body burn fat. Even when you do exercise, the results are not very spectacular, as most people were able to lose just one pound per week.

9) You are not busy enough. This doesn't necessarily mean training, it can mean something else. During fasting, you might be tempted to think of food and it's very hard to resist the temptation of eating something. That's why you definitely need to stay away from the kitchen, or from any refrigerator or plate with food during the fasting period. Keeping your mind and body busy is what can get you through this procedure easily.

10) You abuse caffeine. If you have a very stressful lifestyle and you have your job to thank for this, then probably consuming coffee all the time is something very common for you. You have to get rid of this habit during intermittent fasting, as you will need to stick to just 2 cups of coffee per day, with no sugar or anything else added. It goes without saying that you don't have to drink energy drinks, they have too many calories and are literally poison for your body. One of the purposes of intermittent fasting is to generate energy by burning fats, whether it's the fat tissue or dietary fat. The body is perfectly capable of producing its own energy, so you don't have to drink too much coffee, black tea, energy drinks, or any other kind of drink high in caffeine.

11) You are afraid of experiencing hunger. If you are asking yourself, why I should experience hunger, then this is not the right attitude for IF. "Hunger is a totally normal and natural part of life. Your

muscles won't waste away. You will not die from fasting for 16-20 hours. Your body can survive extreme conditions. Some studies even show that going through stints without food can benefit health. *Short term* deprivation doesn't cause the body to break down muscle and go into 'freak out' mode and gobble up muscle tissue."[27]

27 Michal, Anthony. "9 Common Intermittent Fasting Mistakes." 26 Oct. 2017, anthonymychal.com/intermittent-fasting-mistakes/.

Chapter 12:
Mindset and Tips

I think we can all agree that intermittent fasting is not an easy lifestyle to adapt to, and is definitely not for everyone, even though some are physically fit and healthy enough to try it. Everyone who tries to follow an IF program should be very determined and ambitious. You need to have the right attitude in order to make this procedure work for you. As you already know, mindset is a collection of thoughts and opinions which are reflected in your attitude.

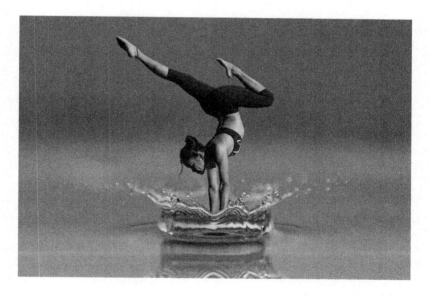

The power of will can get you through this process, regardless of the hardship you experience during IF. After all, intermittent fasting is more of self-discipline and a lifestyle, so it's not something you should only stick to it for a few weeks. There is science behind this procedure, so it's not magic or "voodoo." Every benefit of it can be backed up by science, so if you follow the rules of it, you will most likely experience most of the benefits yourself.

The modern diet includes too much processed food. There are several issues with this type of food. It's unhealthy, it's very calorie dense (so it's high in calories), has little to no nutritional value and it will only keep the hunger away for a very limited amount of time. It causes addiction, as you will need to eat more (and repeatedly), in order to feel satisfied again, but while you are trying to achieve satiety, you are stuffing yourself with carbs (which contain a high amount of glucose).

The main purpose of fasting is to get your body in the fasted state. That's when the magic is happening, so that's when the fat burning process starts. The fasted state can only start 12 hours after your last meal, and this can be very challenging, especially if you are a person who likes to eat a lot and can't go without food for that long. This is when your brain comes into play, as this is the organ capable of not only ignoring or controlling the hunger feelings, but also your actions. So the brain will need to impose the food restrictions for the fasting period. There are several tips to help you go more easily through the intermittent fasting process. Below you can find a list of the most useful tips for achieving this:

1) Stick to shorter fasting periods. As there are several programs to fast, you should first try the ones with a shorter fasting window. This is how you can get used to fasting. You can try daily fasting, or fasting just once or twice per week. You can choose to fast for 16 hours (for the daily Leangains program) or 24 hours (for the Eat-Stop-Eat program or the 5:2 method, i.e., 5 days of normal feeding associated with 2 days of fasting). Trying to fast for more than 24 hours, like 48, 72 and even more hours, is not something that can be done by everyone. "Longer fast periods increase your

risk of problems associated with fasting. This includes dehydration, irritability, mood changes, fainting, hunger, a lack of energy and being unable to focus. The best way to avoid these side effects is to stick to shorter fasting periods of up to 24 hours — especially when you're just starting out. If you want to increase your fasting period to more than 72 hours, you should seek medical supervision."[28]

2) Eat small amounts of food on your fast days. If you are on a daily fasting program, you will need to avoid any calorie consumption during the fasting window, but you will also need to lower the calorie intake for the feeding window. That's why you need to eat nutrient-dense food, so as natural as you can. Most processed food is very low on nutrients and high on calories, so the more natural you eat, the more nutritional value you will get. If you are using the Alternate Day Fast program, this one allows you to consume around 20% of your daily calorie consumption, from a normal feeding day. This method will lower the chances of hunger, dizziness and fatigue, side effects which are usually associated with intermittent fasting.

3) Proper hydration is a must. During intermittent fasting you should only consume water, tea or coffee (without anything added). If you don't hydrate yourself properly, you can experience headaches, dry mouth and also fatigue. The normal fluid intake is around 2 liters per day. However, around 20-30% of the necessary fluids come from your food, but it's not a mandatory rule. You can drink as much as your body demands. "As you meet some of your daily fluid needs through food, you can get dehydrated while fasting. To

---

28 West, Helen. "How to Fast Safely: 10 Helpful Tips." *Healthline*, Healthline Media, 2 Jan. 2019, www.healthline.com/nutrition/how-to-fast#section1.

prevent this, listen to your body and drink when thirsty."[29] Water can also be used to alleviate the feeling of hunger.

4) Meditation and walks can help with IF. When you are feeling hungry or bored, taking long walks or meditating can do the trick and help you get through the fasting period more smoothly. You definitely don't want to think of food, so you need to keep your mind busy through meditation, or you need to stay away from any source of food. Reading a book, listening to music or taking a bath can also help. This is how you can fast for days.

5) Don't feast if you plan to break the fast. There couldn't be a worse way to end the intermittent fasting program than breaking it with a huge meal. After a period during which you trained your body to run on a small number of calories, your stomach and digestive system are no longer used to processing a larger amount of food. So, if you want to feel tired and bloated, then go ahead and eat a copious amount of food. Naturally, a calorie bomb will prevent you from achieving any weight loss goals. One of the main ideas behind IF is the calorie deficit: during this program, you will burn more calories than you consume. Breaking a fast should be just like when one starts the program, you will need to ease into it. Therefore, if you want to break the fast you will need to progressively increase your calorie intake until you are at the optimum level, or what is considered a normal level of calorie consumption. If you do want to quit practicing intermittent fasting, that's your call, but I would highly recommend continuing exercising at the very least.

---

29 West, Helen. "How to Fast Safely: 10 Helpful Tips." *Healthline*, Healthline Media, 2 Jan. 2019, www.healthline.com/nutrition/how-to-fast#section1.

6) Stop fasting if you are not feeling well. One of the main goals of IF is to make you feel better, but there are some side effects to it, like hunger, dizziness or headaches. If you fast for a longer period, you shouldn't keep on fasting regardless of how you feel. Therefore, if you are experiencing any of the symptoms above in an intense manner, you will need to stop immediately. You may experience these side effects if you fast for a longer period, like more than 24 hours. To limit such disadvantages, you might want to limit your fasting period to 24 hours. Remember, intermittent fasting is not for everyone, especially the ones with longer fasting periods. Even the Alternate Day Fast, which includes a fasting window of 36 hours, suggests some calorie intake during fasting. If you start to feel ill or faint, it's always handy to keep a snack at hand. If intermittent fasting makes you feel ill, and you are starting to feel concerned regarding your health, then you need to stop fasting immediately. "Some signs that you should stop your fast and seek medical help include tiredness or weakness that prevents you from carrying out daily tasks, as well as unexpected feelings of sickness and discomfort."[30]

7) Make sure you consume enough protein. When people think of losing weight, they are thinking of burning fat, so they are referring to fat loss. Almost nobody wants to lose muscle mass. There are a few tricks to keeping or even growing muscle mass during IF, and one of them is consuming enough proteins. It's said that the body requires a certain amount of proteins to maintain its muscle mass. Intermittent fasting is a procedure of calorie deficit, which can lead to muscle loss, in addition to fat loss. Fasting days will definitely

30 West, Helen. "How to Fast Safely: 10 Helpful Tips." *Healthline*, Healthline Media, 2 Jan. 2019, www.healthline.com/nutrition/how-to-fast#section1.

not have too many proteins, but there are some programs like the Alternate Day Fast which allow you to have a small calorie intake. You can associate that snack with a protein shake or bar, just to make sure your body has enough proteins to preserve its muscle mass. Consuming food supplements like protein bars or shakes can be an excellent method to use to manage hunger. There are some studies which show that consuming approximately 30% of your meal's calories from protein can lead to a decrease in your appetite.

8) You will need to eat plenty of whole foods during non-fasting days. "Most people who fast are trying to improve their health. Even though fasting involves abstaining from food, it's still important to maintain a healthy lifestyle on days when you are not fasting. Healthy diets based on whole foods are linked to a wide range of health benefits, including a reduced risk of cancer, heart disease, and other chronic illnesses. You can make sure your diet remains healthy by choosing whole foods like meat, fish, eggs, vegetables, fruits, and legumes when you eat."[31]

9) You may need to consume supplements. Food restriction also means nutrient deprivation, so you will not get all the nutrients from your food such as minerals, vitamins and of course the required macronutrients like proteins and healthy fats. Also, consuming fewer calories during the feeding window will definitely not cover your nutritional needs. Protein bars or shakes may not be the only supplements you will need to take, as your body could lack iron, calcium, and vitamins like B12. This is why is important to take multivitamin supplements, to make sure your body will not lack any mineral or vitamin. The best way to assimilate them is

---

31 West, Helen. "How to Fast Safely: 10 Helpful Tips." *Healthline*, Healthline Media, 2 Jan. 2019, www.healthline.com/nutrition/how-to-fast#section1.

from your own food, by having a very well-balanced diet (The Mediterranean diet may be the ideal meal plan in this case because of the wide variety of foods it allows for).

10) If you are new to intermittent fasting, make sure you keep your exercises mild, not intense. Once you get used to IF you can try the intensive training to achieve very good results, but if you are new to this way of eating, just take it slow when it comes to exercising. As your body goes through important changes and it's experiencing nutrient deprivation, you may not have the required resources at the moment to train at maximum capacity. You can imagine that people who are water fasting will not be able to exercise properly on their 5th day of fasting. That's why newbies should try low-intensity (at the beginning) exercises, and add more intensity to your training as soon as you get used to intermittent fasting. Walking, yoga and some stretching may be more than enough in the incipient phase. However, probably the most important tip related to working out is to always listen to your body and allow it to rest if it's feeling tired and struggling with exercises during the fasting window. It's highly recommended to work out during your fasting periods, but if you are new to fasting, keep it mild and gentle when it comes to these workouts during this period. When you get used to the IF lifestyle, you can slowly add some more intensity to your training.

11) Try a LCHF (low carb high fat) diet. When you are trying out the intermittent fasting programs, what you eat during the feeding window is important. Remember, the outcome of IF is to train your body to run on fats, so why not make it easier for it to do so? Ketosis is the metabolic state that encourages ketones to be active and break down the fats. These fats can come from your body's fat tissue or from the fat you eat. The activity of ketones over fats will generate energy. Speaking of dietary fat, you can get them with a proper LCHF diet like the keto diet (which is probably the most

popular diet nowadays), or the Mediterranean diet. The keto diet replaces the carbs from your standard diet with fats, so you will have a nutrient ratio of approximately 75% fats and 5 - 10% carbs (the rest are proteins). The Mediterranean diet is similar enough to the keto diet, but it doesn't have so much fat, and does allow a few more carb-rich foods. However, the carb level is still low enough for the body to achieve ketosis.

If you follow these tips you will most likely succeed in achieving the best results possible through intermittent fasting. However, as a bonus, here are some extra pieces of advice related to this lifestyle:

1) You will need to decide if it suits you. As you already know, intermittent fasting is not for everyone. Eliminating the people who are not physically fit or healthy enough to follow this lifestyle, it's also up to you to decide if you are eligible for any program of IF. Depending on your lifestyle, types of exercises you prefer and nutritional experience, you should be able to establish if this is for you. Find out the basics first, ask for information from a specialist, then decide if you want to go ahead with it.

2) Ease into it. If you are a newbie, you just heard of intermittent fasting and you are curious enough to try it, you need to start with the easiest possible program for you. You can try the daily fast of the Leangains program, or you can fast for only twice a week with the Eat-Stop-Eat program. See if scheduling your meals could be working wonders for you.

3) Concentrate on what every IF program has to offer, and don't get lost in details. All the intermittent fasting programs can eventually have the same benefits, but not all bodies respond in the same way to these programs. Considering that they all have the same benefits, you may need to try more than one program, until you find the right fit for you.

4) Remember to stay flexible. Flexibility, in this case, means to be able to easily switch from one program to another if you don't find a particular one delivering the results you expected.

5) Know yourself. Intermittent fasting is also about self-discovery, not just self-discipline. You can find out what your body's limits are and how it reacts in different situations (find out how long it takes to feel hunger, but also how it can overcome this situation).

6) Allow it some time to work. This is not a "super" diet promising you to lose 10-20 pounds per week. It takes time for its effects to take place, as this lifestyle mostly prepares your body for the fat-loss process. It's believed that a healthy body can perform better, so it puts health first then fat loss. Most people on intermittent fasting have only lost 1 pound per week, which is very slow from some people's point of view. This procedure is one of the most healthy and sustainable methods in terms of fat loss, but in order to fully experience all the health benefits as well, you will need to let it work and try it for a longer period of time.

7) You may experience ups and downs. Not everything with this procedure is "milk and honey." There are some ups and downs with it, just like everything else in life. Keep an open mind and don't freak out when you experience the downs. This is the only way you can focus on achieving the ups.

8) Set the right expectations, so think what exactly you want to achieve from doing this procedure. Intermittent fasting can be considered a very good way to:

- "go deeper into the psychological and physical experience of true hunger
- learn the difference between 'head hunger' and 'body hunger'
- learn not to fear hunger
- improve insulin sensitivity and re-calibrate your body's use of stored fuel

- respect the process and privilege of eating
- learn more about your own body;
- lose fat, *if* you are careful about it
- take a break from the work of food prep and the obligation to eat."[32].

9) "Respect your body cues. Pay attention to what your body tells you. This includes:

1. drastic changes in appetite, hunger, and satiety – including food cravings
2. sleep quality
3. energy levels and athletic performance
4. mood and mental/emotional health
5. immunity
6. blood profile
7. hormonal health
8. how you look"[33]

32 Berardi, John, et al. "All About Intermittent Fasting, Chapter 11." *Precision Nutrition*, www.precisionnutrition.com/intermittent-fasting/appendix-b-tips-and-tricks.
33 Berardi, John, et al. "All About Intermittent Fasting, Chapter 11." *Precision Nutrition*, www.precisionnutrition.com/intermittent-fasting/appendix-b-tips-and-tricks.

Conclusion

Is it really surprising for anyone out there why people nowadays are feeling so sick and are so vulnerable to diseases? Why we are experiencing these major issues when everything should be all about hygiene when it comes to food? How come people who lived 100 years ago didn't experience these issues we are experiencing today? These are all questions we should ask ourselves. The answer lies with the food we consume today.

As most of the food we consume today is processed, and it's far from being in a natural state, we can only think that this food is having harmful effects on our bodies. By harmful effects I mean obesity, heart, lung, liver, kidney and stomach diseases, diabetes, Alzheimer's and Parkinson's disease, and also different types of cancer. More than 70% of the diseases we know today are caused by processed food and high carbs concentration. In fact, processed food has killed more people than cigarettes, drugs, and alcohol put together.

What we think is natural food is not natural at all, so it has been replaced with the term "organic food." Let's think about it, as agriculture uses chemical fertilizers and pesticides on fruits, vegetables, and crops. Animals are being with concentrated food to grow at an incredible rate before they are slaughtered for meat. All of them are ending out in our plate, and the concentrates, fertilizers, pesticides and other chemical compounds used on the animals and fruits or veggies will find a way to affect our internal organs, especially the liver. What we think of as natural food is in fact poisoned food. Organic food is really hard to find. However, the main problem of today's nutrition is processed food and its abundance. As this is the most common type of food sold by supermarkets and fast-food chains, it's no wonder that we are so exposed to it. The modern day lifestyle is encouraging the consumption of such food, which is only calorie dense, and it has little to no nutritional value.

The daily schedule involves a very stressful job, with plenty of tasks during the day and strict deadlines, but also no time to have a proper meal. That's why people are eating fast food and all kinds of unhealthy snacks like chips. The result is simply frightening, as more and more people are facing the risk of becoming overweight or have diabetes. But this is just the tip of the iceberg. People are becoming aware of this issue, but they still consume this kind of food, probably because it's the cheapest. They are trying all sorts of diets and meal plans, most of them promising amazing results (but not delivering). You can understand the frustration of trying something incredibly radical, without having the results you expect, or even having catastrophic results that impact your health.

If you are still looking for the solution to obesity and many other medical conditions, look no further! Intermittent fasting may be the healthiest and most sustainable method to lose weight, but also to heal yourself from common illnesses caused by an excess of carbs. Also, it can prevent or even reverse some diseases or conditions. This way of eating has several programs you can try, according to your needs and possibilities. They can all provide the same benefits.

Intermittent fasting is not a way of eating that was invented or discovered recently, as it was practiced by humans for thousands of years. Since food was scarce back then, humans were required to hunt, fish or pick vegetables and fruits in order to survive. They never knew when their next meal was going to be and sometimes it took more than a few days to have the next meal. The prehistoric humans were a lot stronger, faster and more agile than modern-day humans, and this involuntary fasting had something to do with it, but also the quality of the food they had back then, as everything they consumed was natural.

Fasting was a procedure which was practiced for religious purposes for a long time, but nowadays it's starting to become more popular, as more and more people are discovering its benefits. It's better to combine intermittent fasting with physical exercise and the keto diet, to maximize (and also to speed up the occurrence of) its beneficial effects. The 3 of these can form the "health triad" or the "Holy Trinity of a healthy lifestyle." It may sound a bit much, but trust me, after experiencing the benefits of them you will come to see that its reputation is not misplaced. So, what are you waiting for? Go out there are experience the benefits of IF for yourself today!

Bibliography

1. Berardi, John, et al. "All About Intermittent Fasting, Chapter 11." *Precision Nutrition,* www.precisionnutrition.com/intermittent-fasting/appendix-b-tips-and-tricks.

2. Fung, Jason. "Autophagy – a Cure for Many Present-Day Diseases?" *Diet Doctor*, 19 Dec. 2017, www.dietdoctor.com/autophagy-cure-many-present-day-diseases.

3. Fung, Jason, and Andreas Eenfeldt. "Intermittent Fasting for Beginners – The Complete Guide – Diet Doctor." *Diet Doctor*, 21 May 2019, www.dietdoctor.com/intermittent-fasting/.

4. George, Lesley. "Intermittent Fasting And Muscle Gain: Go To Guide To Fasting Like A Pro • Shapezine - Digital Health & Fitness Tracking Blog." *Shapezine - Digital Health & Fitness Tracking Blog*, 10 July 2018, shapescale.com/blog/health/intermittent-fasting-muscle-gain/.

5. Gunnars, Kris. "How Many Calories Should You Eat Per Day to Lose Weight?" *Healthline*, Healthline Media, 6 July 2018, www.healthline.com/nutrition/how-many-calories-per-day#section1.

6. Jarreau, Paige, and Essential Information. "The 5 Stages of Intermittent Fasting." *LIFE Apps | LIVE and LEARN*, 26 Feb. 2019, lifeapps.io/fasting/the-5-stages-of-intermittent-fasting/.

7. Land, S. (2018). *Metabolic autophagy.* Independently Published,

8. Lefave, Samantha. "8 Major Mistakes People Make When Intermittent Fasting." *What's Good by V*, 31 Jan. 2019, whatsgood.vitaminshoppe.com/intermittent-fasting-mistakes/.

9. Levy, Jillian. "Benefits of Autophagy, Plus How to Induce It." *Dr. Axe*, 4 Sept. 2018, draxe.com/benefits-of-autophagy/.

10. Long, Yun Chau, and Juleen R Zierath. "AMP-Activated Protein Kinase Signaling in Metabolic Regulation." *The Journal of Clinical Investigation*, American Society for Clinical Investigation, 3 July 2006, www.ncbi.nlm.nih.gov/pmc/articles/PMC1483147/.

11. Matus, Mizpah. *Alternate Day Diet*, www.freedieting.com/alternate-day-diet.

12. Michal, Anthony. "9 Common Intermittent Fasting Mistakes." *Anthony Mychal*, 26 Oct. 2017, anthonymychal.com/intermittent-fasting-mistakes/

13. "NCI Dictionary of Cancer Terms." *National Cancer Institute*, www.cancer.gov/publications/dictionaries/cancer-terms/def/mtor.

14. Spritzler, Franziska, and Andreas Eenfeldt. "What Is Ketosis? Is It Safe? – Diet Doctor." *Diet Doctor*, 22 Mar. 2019, www.dietdoctor.com/low-carb/ketosis.

15. West, Helen. "How to Fast Safely: 10 Helpful Tips." *Healthline*, Healthline Media, 2 Jan. 2019, www.healthline.com/nutrition/how-to-fast#section1.

Printed in Great Britain
by Amazon